Department of Health

Report on Health and Social Subjects

43

The Nutrition of Elderly People

Report of the Working Group on the Nutrition of Elderly People
of the Committee on Medical Aspects of Food Policy

London: HMSO

Preface

The proportion of people of pensionable age in this country has been increasing steadily and now represents nearly one in five of the total population. The vast majority of the younger people in this group can look forward to many years of active and enjoyable life and several will remain fit into extreme old age. The right diet contributes to the maintenance of health and wellbeing and it is important that elderly people share in the increasing knowledge about how to maintain health through good nutrition.

In 1990, my predecessor, Sir Donald Acheson, asked Professor Malcolm Hodkinson to chair an expert Working Group of the Committee on Medical Aspects of Food Policy (COMA) to review the nutrition of elderly people. It had been 20 years since COMA last examined the subject and the base of scientific knowledge had enlarged.

The needs of such a heterogeneous group cannot easily be covered in a single report and I am very grateful to Professor Hodkinson and the members of the Working Group for accepting the challenge. I believe that this report will influence nutrition and dietetic practice across a wide spectrum of society, not least in the choices that individual elderly people make about their diet, their physical activity and how much they go out of doors. Above all, I foresee that this Report will stimulate research in this field. It is disappointing that all too often the work of the Group was constrained by lack of data. I am therefore grateful that the Report also makes recommendations about what may be the more fruitful lines of investigation.

Dr Kenneth Calman
Chairman Committee on Medical Aspects of Food Policy

Contents

Committee on Medical Aspects of Food Policy Working Group on the Nutrition of Elderly People

Chairman

Professor H M Hodkinson — Department of Geriatric Medicine, University College and Middlesex School of Medicine, University College, London.

Members

Dr E J Bassey — Department of Physiology and Pharmacology, University of Nottingham, Nottingham.

Professor J Grimley Evans — Division of Geriatric Medicine, Nuffield Department of Clinical Medicine, University of Oxford, Oxford.

Dr R M Francis — Department of Medicine (Geriatrics), Newcastle General Hospital, Newcastle upon Tyne.

Professor O F W James — Department of Medicine (Geriatrics), University of Newcastle upon Tyne, Newcastle upon Tyne.

Professor W P T James — Rowett Research Institute, Aberdeen.

Dr K E Jones — Head of Professional Development (Nursing), Seacroft Hospital, Leeds.

Dr A J Thomas — Plymouth General Hospital, Plymouth.

Observers

Dr J G Ablett — Department of Health, London.

Dr I Higginson — Department of Health, London.

Miss A F Robertson — Department of Health, London.

Mr R W Wenlock	Department of Health, London.
Dr M J Wiseman	Department of Health, London.
Dr J Woolfe	Ministry of Agriculture, Fisheries and Food, London.

Secretariat

Dr P C Clarke (Medical)	Department of Health, London.
Mrs J Caro (Administrative)	Department of Health, London.
Mrs E Lohani (Administrative)	Department of Health, London.

Acknowledgements

The Working Group invited submissions of evidence and wishes to record with gratitude contributions from the following individuals and groups:

Professor D J P Barker	MRC Environmental Epidemiology Unit, University of Southampton.
Dr V W Bunker	Department of Clinical Biochemistry, Portsmouth Polytechnic.
Mrs R I Coupland	Orpington, Kent.
Ms J Fenton	Springfield Psychogeriatric Hospital, Wandsworth, London.
Ms E McEwen	Age Concern, London.
Mr G Meteau	Worthing, Sussex.
Ms P Taylor	Selly Oak Hospital, Birmingham.
Dr J D Walter	British Society for the Study of Prosthetic Dentistry, Guy's Hospital, London.

1. Summary of the report and recommendations

Summary of the report

1.1 The Working Party on the Nutrition of Elderly People recommends that the majority of people aged 65 years or more should adopt, where possible, similar patterns of eating and lifestyle to those advised for maintaining health in younger adults. Physical activity improves muscle tone and power, and leads to higher energy expenditure. A diet which provides an adequate intake of all nutrients can more easily be obtained if the energy intake remains at a level close to that recommended for younger adults.

1.2 The recommendations from the Panel on Dietary Reference Values of the Committee on Medical Aspects of Food Policy (COMA) are endorsed[1]. The Working Party recommends that elderly people should reduce dietary intakes of fat and simple sugars and increase intakes of starchy foods, non-starch polysaccharides and vitamin D. Where there are no data on which to base advice, lines for research are recommended.

1.3 An area of particular concern was the impact of illness and disability on nutritional status in this age group. There are few data as to energy and nutrient requirements in health in this population group, but those in acute illness, chronic illness or disability are virtually unknown. There was concern that low body weight is so common a finding in chronically ill or disabled old people. This suggested that energy intakes may be inadequate, particularly among very disabled old people being cared for in institutions where low weights are particularly common. The need for research in this area seemed particularly great especially in addressing the possibility of "institutional starvation". A related problem was that of nutrient density of the diet. Total energy intakes may become so low in chronically sick or disabled old people that, unless the nutrient density of the diet is unusually high, adequate intakes of specific nutrients are very unlikely to be achieved. Detailed knowledge of the requirements for this sub-group of the elderly population for specific nutrients is of considerable practical importance and needs more detailed study.

1.4 Many of the anthropometric measurements used in nutritional surveys were derived for younger adults. Those based on the measurement of height are of questionable value when used in elderly populations. Loss of height due to disc degeneration or vertebral collapse may make it difficult, or indeed impossible, to measure height in disabled old people who are unable to stand unaided. Even if measurable, skeletal height may not be a good index of skeletal size in these circumstances. Alternatives to height measurement need evaluation.

1

1.5 Finally, there needs to be greater awareness of the importance of good nutrition for maintaining the health of elderly people and of its contribution to recovery from illness. Nutrition education and health promotion programmes should include this population group.

1.6 **Recommendations of the Working Group on Nutrition of Elderly People**

The recommendations listed below are discussed in the relevant chapters.

Recommendations to maintain good nutritional status in elderly people

1. The Working Group endorsed the recommendations for people aged over 50 years in the Government publication *Dietary Reference Values for Food Energy and Nutrients for the United Kingdom*.[1] (Chapter 3)

2. Recommendations for dietary energy intakes of elderly people should tend to the generous, except for those who are obese. (Chapter 4)

3. Elderly people should derive their dietary intakes from a diet containing a variety of nutrient dense foods (Chapter 4).

4. An active life style, with prompt resumption after episodes of intercurrent illness, is recommended as contributing in several ways to good health. (Chapter 4)

5. Steps should be taken to increase the awareness by health professionals of the importance of both overweight and underweight in elderly people. (Chapter 5)

6. For the majority of elderly people, the same recommendations concerning the dietary intake of non-milk extrinsic sugars apply as for the younger adult population. (Chapter 6)

7. Intakes of non-starch polysaccharides comparable to those recommended for the general population are advised for most elderly people. Foods with high phytate content, especially raw bran, should be avoided or used sparingly. (Chapter 6)

8. The statutory fortification of yellow fats other than butter with vitamin A and D should continue, and manufacturers are encouraged to fortify other fat spreads voluntarily. (Chapter 7)

9. Elderly people should be encouraged to increase their dietary intakes of vitamin C. (Chapter 7)

10. Adequate intakes of vitamin C need to be ensured for elderly people who are dependent on institutional catering. (Chapter 7).

2

11. Elderly people, in common with those of all ages, should be advised to eat more fresh vegetables, fruit, and whole grain cereals. (Chapter 7)

12. Elderly people should be encouraged to adopt diets which moderate their plasma cholesterol levels. (Chapter 9)

13. There should be encouragement of elderly people to consume oily fish and to maintain physical activity in order to reduce the risk of thrombosis. (Chapter 9)

14. The Working Group endorsed the WHO recommendation that 6 g/d sodium chloride would be a reasonable average intake for the elderly population in the UK, and recommends that the present average dietary salt intakes be reduced to meet this level. (Chapter 9)

15. The calcium intakes of elderly people in the UK should be monitored. (Chapter 10)

16. Doorstep deliveries of milk for elderly people should be maintained. (Chapter 10)

17. All elderly people should be encouraged to expose some skin to sunlight regularly during the months May to September. (Chapter 10)

18. If adequate exposure to sunlight is not possible, vitamin D supplementation should be considered especially during the winter and early spring. (Chapter 10)

19. Health professionals should be made aware of the impact of nutritional status on the development of and recovery from illness. (Chapter 12)

20. Health professionals should be aware of the often inadequate food intake of elderly people in institutions. (Chapter 12)

21. Assessment of nutritional status should be a routine aspect of history taking and clinical examination when an elderly person is admitted to hospital. (Chapter 12)

Recommendations for investigation and research

22. Further studies are needed to quantify energy requirements for elderly people which take individual health status into account with particular emphasis on those who are thin. (Chapter 4)

23. Techniques to measure energy expenditure including the doubly labelled water method should be evaluated further in elderly people. (Chapter 4)

24. Further research should validate the best anthropometric methods for field work with elderly people. (Chapter 5)

25.   Demispan measurements should be extended to all nutritional surveys of elderly people and some of younger adults in order to assess its relationship to other measures of skeletal size and to parameters of health. (Chapter 5)

26.   The prognostic significance of body mass index and other anthropometric measures in a British population of elderly people should be clarified. (Chapter 5)

27.   Further research should be done to determine with more precision the protein requirements of elderly people. (Chapter 6)

28.   The micronutrient intakes of elderly people in the UK need to be determined. (Chapter 7)

29.   The micronutrient requirements of the elderly population need to be determined more accurately. (Chapter 7)

30.   The clinical features of deficiency of vitamins from the B group especially thiamin, vitamin B_{12} and folate need to be investigated. (Chapter 7)

31.   Better biochemical indices of vitamin C status need to be developed. (Chapter 7)

32.   There should be further research to assess magnesium status in ill elderly people, particularly those with cardiac failure. (Chapter 8)

33.   The iron status of elderly people in this country should be determined. (Chapter 8)

34.   Clinical and biochemical markers of both zinc and copper status need to be defined more precisely. (Chapter 8)

35.   Research is needed into the nutritional component to the attainment of peak bone mass. (Chapter 10)

36.   Further studies are needed to determine optimal intakes of calcium for the elderly population. (Chapter 10)

37.   Research is needed on the clinical features of vitamin D deficiency. (Chapter 10)

38.   The relationships between the development of cancer and dietary energy and nutrients should continue to be investigated. (Chapter 11)

39.   Methodologies should be developed for the determination of antioxidant status. (Chapter 11)

40.   The impact of acute and chronic illness on the nutritional requirements of the elderly needs comprehensive study. (Chapter 12)

41.   Parameters of nutritional status with prognostic significance in ill elderly patients should be determined. (Chapter 12)

42.   Effective methods of ensuring adequate nutrition need to be developed and evaluated, especially for elderly people in hospital or institutions. (Chapter 12)

2. Introduction

2.1 Good nutrition contributes to the health of elderly people and to their ability to recover from illness. The Committee on Medical Aspects of Food Policy (COMA) convened a Working Group in 1990 to examine the available data on the nutrition of elderly people. Their report updates an earlier one from COMA in 1970 (para 3.1.1)[2]. The 1990 Working Group reviewed and assessed available scientific evidence and drew conclusions where possible. No new research was commissioned.

2.2 Terms of reference of the Working Group and meetings

"To review the nutrition of elderly people and to make a report".

The dietetic implications of achieving good nutrition were considered where they contribute to the development of a nutrition policy for elderly people. Implementing such a policy successfully requires inter-sectoral collaboration and a multi disciplinary approach and the Working Group considered that proposing detailed dietetic modifications did not fall within its terms of reference. The Working Group met five times. The Department of Health issued a Press Release which invited submissions from interested organisations or individuals. These contributions are acknowledged earlier.

2.3 **Demographic trends** In 1990, thirteen per cent of the male population and nineteen per cent of the female population of England and Wales were aged 65 years or over. Thus, of the total population aged 16 years or over, a little more than one in six were elderly people. By the year 2030 it is predicted that elderly people will account for one in four of the adult population. The sex ratio of men to women in the group aged 65 years or more was 0.67 in 1991. It is predicted that this ratio will increase to 0.72 in 2001 because, although increasing numbers of men are expected to live longer, women over 65 years will also increase in number especially those who are aged over 75 years.

In 1977, some 150,000 people over 65 years were living in residential homes and by 1987 this total had increased to 210,000[3].

2.4 **Definitions** Throughout the Report the generic term used for the population aged 65 years or more is "elderly people".

  i. *Young elderly people* are aged from 65 to 74 years.

  ii. *Older elderly people* are aged 75 years or older.

Institutionalized elderly people live permanently in residential homes, in long stay hospital wards or in nursing homes. *Non-institutionalized elderly people*

6

are *free living* and represent the majority or are *housebound* elderly people who have been unable to leave their house independently for at least three months.

2.5 Abbreviations

g	gram
mg	milligram or 10^{-3}g or one-thousandth of 1g
μg	microgram or 10^{-6}g or one-millionth of 1g
ng	nanogram or 10^{-9}g or one-thousand-millionth of 1g
kg	kilogram or 10^3g or 1000g
mmol	millimol = atomic or molecular weight of element or compound in g $\times 10^{-3}$
kcal	kilocalorie = 10^3 or 1000 calories. A unit used to measure the energy value of food
kJ	kilojoule = 10^3 or 1000 Joules. A unit used to measure the energy value of food 1 kcal = 4.18kJ
1 mJ	megajoule = 10^6J or 1 million Joules
m	metre

3. Background

3.1 Previous nutrition surveys of elderly people in Britain*

3.1.1   The COMA Panel on Nutrition of the Elderly reported in 1970[2]. They reviewed the available information and concluded that the quality of the diet did not change with age but that the quantity tended to decrease. Osteomalacia was identified as an occasional problem. A nutritional survey by geriatricians of patients admitted to hospital had identified a small number of men and women with overt nutritional inadequacy which was usually linked to unfavourable social circumstances or to pre-existing disease.

3.1.2   A more detailed diet and nutrition survey had been started in six towns in England and Scotland in 1967/8 which used dietary recall and diary methods to assess the energy and nutrient intakes. Full information was obtained on 764 elderly people[4]. There was a further study in 1972/3 of 365 surviving people who had participated in the 1967/8 survey and who could be traced[5]. These surveys excluded people in institutional care. Among the findings in 1967/8 were geographical and sex differences in energy and nutrient intakes. Three per cent of those surveyed were diagnosed as having malnutrition and in three-quarters of these cases this was in association with clinical disease. In 1972/3, seven per cent of the group surveyed were considered to be malnourished and this condition was more prevalent in those over 80 years of age. Several medical and social risk factors for malnutrition were identified of which the most important was being housebound. A major conclusion of the survey was that, provided individual elderly people were in good health, their dietary patterns and the foods eaten were no different from what is known about those of younger people. The results of the 1972/3 survey have been used in several sections of the present report because they are the most recent published national nutritional data about elderly people. A further survey of a representative sample of 1000 elderly people was carried out for the COMA Panel on the Elderly in 1973/4 but no report of this study was published.

3.2 The Dietary and Nutritional Survey of British Adults

In 1986/7, 2197 people living in Britain aged 16 to 64 years recorded their weighed dietary intakes for seven days, were measured for height, weight and blood pressure, and provided blood and urine for analysis[6]. This survey provides more up-to date information about the diet of a nationally representative sample of younger adults, and, for the reasons given above, (para 3.1.2) it may also reflect the dietary patterns of elderly people.

---

*Throughout the text the convention is adopted of identifying surveys according to the year of the fieldwork.

3.3 Dietary Reference Values for food energy and nutrients In 1991 the Department of Health published a report from COMA on Dietary Reference Values for the United Kingdom for food energy and for some 40 nutrients[1]. This gives an up-to-date and comprehensive review of knowledge about requirements for energy and each of the nutrients; the macronutrients fat and carbohydrate are considered in this context for the first time[1]. The use of Dietary Reference Values (DRV) supplants the earlier "recommended daily amount" (RDA). The definitions of DRV together with the recommended DRV for the population over 50 years of age for vitamins and minerals are presented in Annex 1, and for energy and other nutrients in the relevant sections. These scientific arguments are not generally repeated in this report on elderly people. Nutritional reviews concerning elderly people are especially constrained by lack of data. Where nutrients are not addressed in this report, it can be assumed that the Working Group found no information additional to that already examined by COMA in formulating the report on DRV.

3.4 Recommendation

1. The Working Group endorsed the recommendations for people aged over 50 years in the Government publication *Dietary Reference Values for Food Energy and Nutrients for the United Kingdom*.

4. Energy and physical activity

4.1 Dietary energy requirements

4.1.1 The COMA Panel on DRV based its figures for the Estimated Average Requirement (EAR) for energy for population groups aged 60 years or more on a standard value of 1.5 × Basal Metabolic Rate (BMR)[1] (Table 4.1). This was adopted for several reasons including the paucity of data on energy intake and expenditure as well as the diversity of physical activity patterns in this group of the population. The Panel also wished to avoid an incremental approach for the group of people with very low activity levels including some of those in institutions, especially bedridden people. If the EAR for elderly people is derived incrementally, it will be so low in some cases that achieving an adequate diet from normal food becomes impossible (para 4.5.3).

Table 4.1: *Estimated Average Daily Requirements (EAR) for Energy*[1]

Age (years)	EAR mJ (kcal)/d	
	males	females
19–50	10.60 (2550)	8.10 (1940)
51–59	10.60 (2550)	8.00 (1900)
60–64	9.93 (2380)	7.99 (1900)
65–74	9.71 (2330)	7.96 (1900)
75 +	8.77 (2100)	7.61 (1810)

4.1.2 Other expert groups have tried to be more precise. The FAO/WHO/UNU Expert Consultation (1985) identified several determinants of energy status when defining the energy requirement of an individual as the level of energy intake from food that will balance expenditure when the individual has a body size and composition and level of physical activity consistent with long-term good health; and that will allow for the maintenance of economically necessary and socially desirable physical activity[7]. This prescriptive approach was not adopted in its entirety by COMA for the reasons given above.

4.2 Energy expenditure

4.2.1 Both maintaining basic bodily functions, for example, keeping warm, and physical activity require energy. Information on energy expenditure in elderly people is very limited. Data collected before 1970 has been collated from several studies[8]. A more recent study in Holland reported lower mean energy expenditures than those observed in the studies twenty years earlier (Table 4.2)[9].

4.2.2 Techniques using doubly labelled water have been developed to measure the total energy expenditure in free living people. The theoretical accuracy of the method is reported to be about 5 per cent in adults[10]. Water enriched with molecules in which both the hydrogen and the oxygen atoms are stable isotopes (deuterium and ^{18}O) is ingested. The hydrogen labels the water pool and the oxygen labels both the water and the carbon dioxide produced from metabolic processes. A comparison of the rates of dilution of the two isotopes from the body, assessed over time in body fluids such as urine or plasma, can be used to estimate carbon dioxide production and so, as in classical indirect calorimetry, total energy expenditure[11]. There is debate about whether both labels equilibrate with the same water pool, and assumptions have to be made, for example about respiratory quotient and insensible losses of water through the skin. The method, which is non-invasive and simple for the subject, appears particularly suitable for elderly people (para 12.3.2) and should be validated in this population.

Table 4.2: *Daily energy expenditure in groups of elderly people*

	Durnin 1985[8] several countries		Fredrix et al 1990[9] Holland	
Sex	M	F	M	F
Number	ns	ns	18	22
Age (year)	"elderly retired"	60–69 (living alone)	63 ± 8*	66 ± 7*
Mean energy expenditure kcal (mJ)/d	2330(9.7)	1990(8.3)	1733 ± 205*	1330 ± 155*
Range kcal (mJ)/d	1750–2810 (7.3–11.8)	1490–2140 (6.2–9.0)	(7.3 ± 0.86)	(5.6 ± 0.65)
Mean energy expenditure (kcal/mean kg wt)	ns	ns	21	21

* ± standard deviation
ns not stated

4.3 Basal metabolic rate (BMR)

4.3.1 BMR describes the energy needed per day to maintain vital functions; it increases with body size, particularly with lean body mass, and so it is higher in men than women. The FAO/WHO/UNU Expert Consultation[7] used equations to predict BMR[12]. These equations may be less appropriate for the elderly population, especially older men, because of the small numbers in the study. Additional data have therefore been collected which allow a more precise estimate of current energy requirements and energy balance in an elderly European population (Table 4.3). BMR declines with age in both sexes (Table 4.4). BMR per kg fat-free mass tends to be unchanged with age[13] and it is the fall in total mass of lean tissue with age which determines this decline in absolute BMR.

4.4 Dietary energy intake

4.4.1 The results of cross-sectional surveys of dietary energy intakes of elderly people who are living independently in the community have shown that men consistently consume more food energy than women, even after standardising for body mass. Elderly subjects from USA consume on average more energy than subjects examined in European studies (Table 4.5). The mean dietary energy intakes of adults aged 16–64 years in Britain in 1986 were 10.3 mJ (2450 kcal)/d for men and 7.0 mJ (1680 kcal)/d for women[6]. The European Collaborative Study on Nutrition in the Elderly was conducted in several European countries in 1988/9. There was great variation in energy intakes between individuals within the European countries surveyed and substantial variation between countries[16].

Table 4.3: *Equations for predicting basal metabolic rate (mJ/d) in people aged over 60 years*

	Age group (years)	Equation by weight: W(kg)	Equation by weight: W(kg) height: H(cm)
Male	60–74	0.0499W + 2.930	0.048W + 0.0059H + 2.06
	75 +	0.0350W + 3.434	0.0311W + 0.0141H + 1.40
Female	60–74	0.0386W + 2.875	0.0368W + 0.0153H + 0.65
	75 +	0.0410W + 2.610	0.037W + 0.026H − 1.04

The original data included only 50 men and 38 women over 60 years of age[12]. Data on the European subjects from this group have been collated with data on 101 men aged 60–70 years studied by Durnin, and with unpublished data on 170 men and 180 women supplied by Ferro-Luzzi to prepare the equations in this table.

Table 4.4: *Changes in basal metabolic rate with age*

Age (years)	25	40	59	70	75 +
Male					
Median weight	73	75	73	74	67
BMR (mJ/d)	7.50	7.32	7.16	6.62*	5.78*
Female					
Median weight	58	62	63	63	58
BMR (mJ/d)	6.49	5.73	5.76	5.31*	4.99*

The standard Schofield equations were applied to the 25–59 year old groups and weights from a representative sample of adults in Great Britain in 1980[14]. The new equations from Table 4.3 were used to calculate BMR for elderly subjects using weights from a survey in Nottingham[15].

4.4.2 The DHSS study begun in 1967/8 gives longitudinal data , about energy intakes in elderly people[4]. 365 people were examined in 1967/8 and again five years later; the average energy intakes had fallen from 9.4 to 9.0 mJ (2235 to 2151 kcal)/d for men and from 7.2 to 6.8 mJ (1711 to 1636 kcal)/d for women[5]. A similar trend for energy intakes to fall with age over a five year period was observed in a study of 269 elderly people in Gothenberg, Sweden[17]. The 1986/7 Dietary and Nutritional Survey of British Adults was not longitudinal but comparing the average food energy intakes between age groups suggests a trend towards decreasing energy intakes in older age. The highest average intakes were recorded for men and women under 50 years of age[6].

Table 4.5: *Daily dietary energy intakes in groups of elderly people living in the community**

Year of study and country

	Durnin et al (1961)[18] Scotland		McGandy et al (1966)[19] USA		Borgstrom et al (1979)[20] Sweden		DHSS (1979)[5] Britain		Uauy et al (1978)[21] USA		Bunker et al (1989)[22] Southampton		Loenen et al (1990)[23] Holland	
Sex	M	F	M	F	M	F	M	F	M	F	M	F	M	F
Number	9	21	50	37	17	20	169	196	6	6	11	13	237	223
Age (yrs)	64–77	60–69	67–74	77–99	67–73	69–97	69–90	68–74	70–84	63–77	70–85	69–85	65–79	65–79
Mean energy intake (kcal)	2055	1894	2297	2093	2050	1600	2151	1636	2325	1904	2071	1571	2440	1910
Mean daily energy intake (kcal)/mean wt (kg)	30	31	30	29	27	23	33	28	31	28	30	25	32	28

*See also Table 12.1

13

4.4.3 The surveys of elderly people in Great Britain in 1967/8 and 1972/3 concluded that they ate similar foods to those in the diets of younger people and therefore the lower energy intakes almost certainly reflect a lower consumption of food. The decline in energy intake was less marked when total dietary energy was expressed per kilogram body weight because of the declining weight with age associated with loss of muscle mass (para 4.3). Although a proportion of elderly people, especially those who are very elderly, appear to remain in good health while consuming a declining quantity of food and losing weight very slowly over several years, concerns have arisen that energy intakes may be so low as not to support an adequate intake of all essential nutrients. Subgroups of the elderly population who suffer chronic disability or repeated illnesses and who have very low energy intakes are particularly at risk of nutritional inadequacy (Chapter 12).

4.5 Effect of declining energy intake on the nutritional adequacy of the diet

4.5.1 Providing an adequate nutrient intake for elderly people becomes dietetically difficult once body weight and physical activity start to decline. Even if energy intake needs are maintained at EAR levels of 1.5 × BMR (Table 4.1), as the average weight of the population falls, men and women need to obtain the same nutrient intakes when they are over 75 years of age despite reductions of BMR of 17 per cent and 6 per cent respectively when compared with younger adults (Table 4.4).

4.5.2 Many elderly people spend only about 1 hour per day on their feet so that a value of 1.3 × BMR often applies. On this basis, elderly people who continue to consume food energy equivalent to 1.5 × BMR may become obese[24]. Conversely, even if in energy balance, at 1.3 × BMR, an 80 year old man may, for example, only be eating 7.6 mJ compared with a value of 10.6 mJ when younger. This 28 per cent decline in energy expenditure and intake makes it difficult to allow an appropriate intake of nutrients and non-starch polysaccharides without a substantial change in the diet of elderly men.

4.5.3 Given low body weights and low activity levels, the opportunities for dietary modification to increase nutrient intakes are very limited if the overall food consumption is low. For example, current healthy eating advice is to increase intakes of vegetables, fruit and non-starch polysaccharides. Milk intakes need to be maintained to ensure an adequate amount of calcium. Since a decline in protein intake is not recommended, then an intake of 1 g protein/kg body weight signifies an increase in the protein content of the diet of an 80 year old man from 13.1 per cent of dietary energy where one activity level is 1.5 × BMR, to 15.2 per cent of dietary energy where the activity level becomes 1.3 × BMR. On this basis, the only means of ensuring nutrient intake is to have a low (below 10 per cent) sugar intake. If the energy intake falls by a third with a proportional reduction in the consumption of all food items, then elderly people may be more likely to develop symptoms of constipation. These examples demonstrate the complexity of integrating dietary advice to achieve an adequate diet once elderly people have become underweight and inactive.

4.5.4　There are health benefits for elderly people if they can avoid becoming underweight (para 5.5.1). A diet rich in starchy foods, cereals, vegetables and fruit as the habitual diet of the middle aged before retirement will help to ensure that a diet is maintained in later life which is sufficient to meet requirements as energy intakes decline. Appetite may wane in elderly people especially if they are ill (para 12.2) and dietetic and culinary skills and ingenuity become increasingly important to ensure that elderly people continue to find eating pleasurable.

4.6　Physical activity of elderly people

4.6.1　Current perceptions of the value of exercise for elderly people need to be changed so that it is recognised that a physically active life is beneficial and, barring serious illness, possible well into the eighth decade of life. Physical activity contributes to good physical and psychological health at all ages[25]. For younger adults, periods of sustained vigorous activity may benefit cardiac health. At all ages, the value of simple walking, gentle cycling, swimming or other mild exercise should not be underestimated. As people get older, their desire for physical activity may decline and opportunities diminish. People who are not in paid employment may choose not to go out and this particularly pertains to older elderly people.

4.6.2　The General Household Survey (GHS) is a questionnaire survey based on a sample of the general population resident in private (non-institutional) households in Britain. In 1985 the GHS collected information from 3691 people aged 65 years or over which included questions about participation in physical activities in the previous four weeks. At all ages walking was the most common activity but small numbers of people took part in a variety of physical leisure activities[26] (Table 4.6). In the 60–69 year age group about 70 per cent recorded no outdoor activity in the previous four weeks and this proportion was even higher in the over 70 year age group.

Table 4.6: *Participation rates by British adults in physical activities in the 4 weeks before interview 1985 (per cent)*[26]

| | Age (yrs) | | | | | |
| | Men | | | Women | | |
	30–44	60–69	70+	30–44	60–69	70+
ACTIVITY						
Walking						
2 miles or more	23	23	16	21	20	7
Swimming	3	2	1	3	1	0
Cycling	3	1	1	2	0	0
Keepfit/yoga	–	–	–	8	2	1
At least 1 outdoor activity:						
excluding walking	32	13	7	13	4	2
including walking	45	31	20	29	22	9

4.6.3 A survey of customary activity of elderly people living at home in Nottingham found that the average reported daily time in active pursuits was less than one hour and lower still in those aged 75 years or more (Table 4.7) [27, 15]. A large number of people were relatively inactive although a few were very active. There were weak negative associations with age within the sample in most of the activity variables. Four years later a significant decline in activity levels was found in the 600 survivors.

4.6.4 The energy cost of normal activities has been reported to increase with age for men[8]. In Nottingham, healthy women aged 70 years had a 20 per cent higher energy cost for walking at a standard speed than either men of the same age or younger women[28,29] which rose to 25 per cent when walking a standard distance at their own chosen speed. This increase was attributed to slower speed with a longer duration and a greater body weight as well as reduced efficiency. There was a significantly reduced stride length, possibly due to increased stiffness or reduced confidence in weakened muscles. Women with overt problems such as amputation, arthritis or overweight are likely to experience greater increases in energy cost.

4.6.5 Inactivity associated with a minor illness often leads to loss of muscle tone and mass and thereafter former physical activity levels may never be regained. This stepwise decline is often seen by individuals and their families as inevitable, as in some cases it is. On the other hand, an approach which stimulates continued activity, even vigorous at times, may result in increasing capacity for activity with measurable increase in muscle mass[30,31].

4.7 Recommendations

1. Further studies are needed to quantify energy requirements for elderly people which take individual health status into account with particular emphasis on those who are thin.

2. Techniques to measure energy expenditure including the doubly labelled water method should be evaluated further in elderly people.

3. Recommendations for dietary energy intakes of elderly people should tend to the generous, except for those who are obese.

4. Elderly people should derive their dietary energy intakes from a diet containing a variety of nutrient dense foods.

5. An active life style, with prompt resumption after episodes of intercurrent illness, is recommended as contributing in several ways to good health.

Table 4.7: *Time allocation in Italian*** and English[15] elderly people living at home (hours and minutes per day: mean** values)*

	Women					Men				
Age (yrs)	English			Italian		English			Italian	
	60–69	70–79	80 +	65–74	75 +	60–69	70–79	80 +	65–74	75 +
Sleep	7.24	7.55	8.10	6.59	7.10	7.24	7.55	8.24	7.05	7.23
Rest in bed	1.55	2.24	3.07	1.45	1.56	1.55	1.55	2.50	1.28	1.22
Sitting										
inactive	5.16	5.46	6.28			6.00	6.28	6.44		
active	1.55	2.09	1.55			1.40	1.40	1.40		
Standing										
inactive	0.58	0.43	0.43			1.27	1.12	0.43		
active	0.58	0.43	0.15			2.09	1.55	1.12		
Walking, stairs	0.43	0.43	0.29			1.12	0.58	0.43		
Moving about	4.34	3.36	2.38			2.09	1.55	1.40		
Indoor + outdoor + leisure*				2.04	1.44				2.27	1.60
Walking				0.55	0.26				0.54	0.39
Other activity	<0.15	<0.15	<0.15	0.0	0.0	<0.15	<0.15	0.15	1.0	1.0

*** Unpublished data provided by Professor Ferro Luzzi.

** Some of these data are skewed, so the means are markedly higher than the median values.

* Includes housework, gardening and house maintenance likely to have an energy cost of at least 2 kcal/min, performed for at least 3 minutes continuously with a regularity of at least weekly, sampled over the previous 6 weeks during May—September.

Sampled on the day preceding the interview; only purposeful walking outside the house and garden is included (leisure walking is counted as leisure).

5. Assessment of body size and composition in elderly people: changes with age and significance for health

5.1 There are extensive data on measured external body dimensions such as height and weight, circumferences and skin fold thicknesses for adults aged under 60 years. It is not appropriate to use these normative data at older ages because changes due to ageing affect body shape, size and composition.

5.2 The assessment of skeletal size

5.2.1 *Height* The assessment of skeletal size from height alone is often unsatisfactory for old people because of the frequency of kyphosis, vertebral collapse and loss of disc height. Furthermore, a proportion of elderly people will be unable to stand. Measurement of a segment of the body other than the spine avoids these problems.

5.2.2 *Demispan* Demispan is the measurement from the web between the fingers along the outstretched arm to the sternal notch with the arm in the coronal plane. The wrist is kept in neutral rotation and neutral flexion. Total arm length and total span are reported to change with age considerably less than height[32]. The measurement of demispan has proved satisfactory in the hands of relatively untrained observers. It can be measured seated. Its measurement is socially acceptable and requires only one observer. A stainless steel tape is all that is required to measure the distance between the finger roots, where it is anchored between the subject's middle and ring fingers, and the sternal notch.

5.2.3 *Knee height* This is a short skeletal segment and therefore errors of measurement are relatively larger. It is measured seated which is an advantage for frail individuals, but location of the knee joint space as an anatomical marker is sometimes difficult.

5.3 Body composition in elderly people

5.3.1 *Relative body mass* The relative body mass, or mass in relation to skeletal size, gives an indication of fatness. Body Mass Index (BMI; mass in kg divided by height in m squared) is the most commonly used ratio in younger adults[14]. The published norms assume that lean mass is proportional to skeletal size, and only the fat varies[33]. In assessing fatness in younger adults, BMI correlates with fatness measured using skinfold thickness with an explained variance of about 60 per cent. BMI is only suitable for within-race comparisons and standards for comparison should be specific for ethnic group.

18

5.3.2　BMI is not a valid measure of relative mass in a proportion of the elderly population partly because of the problems of measuring height. Indices have been developed which use demispan measurement instead of height. The "demiquet" is mass divided by demispan squared, and the "mindex" is mass divided by demispan. Ranges of values for these indices in groups of elderly people have been established and are useful to identify those at the extremes of the distribution (see Table 5.1). Those so identified are not necessarily malnourished, but further investigation may be indicated[34].

5.3.3　*Skinfold thickness*　The measurement of skinfold thickness using constant pressure callipers at standard sites on the body provides a cheap and non-invasive assessment of subcutaneous fat. The technique is reliable only in practised hands, with a coefficient of variation of about 6 per cent. In elderly people there are probably changes in skinfold compressibility which have not been adequately described and differences in the proportion of subcutaneous to deep body fat stores, also known to change with age, contribute further variations. Skinfold thickness measurements in elderly people offer only a rough guide to body fatness, and they must be assessed in conjunction with other indicators.

Table 5.1: *Mean values and ranges for weight, demispan and derived ratios in groups of elderly people: Nottingham Activity and Ageing Survey*

	Age range (yrs)	Number	Weight (kg)*	Demispan (cm)*	Demiquet (kg/m²)*	Mindex (kg/m)*
Men	65–74	205	72.5 ± 12.6 (39–114)	81.6 ± 4.05 (71.5–92.7)	108.8 ± 17.2 (68.6–162.6)	
	75–91	153	68.6 ± 11.4 (43–94)	80.4 ± 4.1 (71.5–91.3)	106.0 ± 15.1 (72.0–153.6)	
Women	65–74	257	64.5 ± 13.3 (35–124)	73.8 ± 3.6 (63.3–84.0)		87.3 ± 17.4 (49.9–168)
	75–94	275	59.7 ± 11.6 (35–102)	72.7 ± 3.5 (64.2–84.8)		82.1 ± 15.2 (49.3–86.8)

*Mean values ± 1 standard deviation (and range)
(Taken from Lehmann et al 1991[34])

A randomly selected sample of free living people in Nottingham, evenly divided between the ages 65–74 years and 75 years and over, were used to establish a range of values for weight and skeletal size.

5.3.4　*Body Composition*　There are limitations on the methods based on empirical relations such as the BMI. An alternative approach is to assess different compartments of the body which are related to the fat or to the lean body mass independently; for instance, water or potassium are associated almost, but not quite exclusively, with lean tissue. A distinction must be made between adipose tissue and fat mass since adipose tissue contains about 14 per cent water and 2 per cent protein in addition to fat. Also, there is a fat component to tissues other than adipose tissue. Few methods are entirely satisfactory even in young adults and for elderly people they are even less so. A critical comment on several methods is at Annex 2.

5.3.5   Changes in body mass do not necessarily reflect the accumulation or loss of adipose tissue especially in elderly people. In the UK, body mass tends to increase through middle age due to an accumulation of fat, and thereafter it declines in association with, among other changes, loss of lean tissue[35,36]. Longitudinal studies confirm the loss of lean tissue but estimates of the rate of loss vary[37]. The effect of a proportional reduction in lean body mass will give rise to an underestimate of fatness as reflected in the relative weight. On the other hand, oedema which may be present in the elderly, results in an over-estimate of fatness.

5.4   Overweight

5.4.1   BMI values for the subjects in the 1972/3 DHSS survey of the nutrition of elderly people are shown in Table 5.2. Using this index there were fewer overweight and more underweight people in the 75 year and over age group than in the group aged 65 to 74 years. The 1972/3 DHSS survey of elderly people also examined the relationship between obesity and disease[5]. No excess of hyperten-sion or diabetes was found among those considered to be obese by the examining physician. This may have arisen because susceptible individuals had died or, in part, due to difficulty in appropriately defining obesity. Excess fat might be expected to embarrass a failing cardiorespiratory system, for instance in those with heart failure or chronic bronchitis. There is a higher prevalence of osteoarthritis of the knees in overweight elderly women and some studies have reported a similar relationship in men[38]. It is not desirable for elderly people to be overweight because any additional physical burden is likely to restrict activity levels with a resulting reduction in muscle mass. The social and psychological benefits of going out of doors and meeting people will also be reduced.

5.5   Underweight

5.5.1   The DHSS survey of 1972/73 found that 18.3 per cent of elderly men and 11.5 per cent of elderly women were thin defined as a body mass index of less than 20 (Table 5.2)[5]. In the 1986/7 survey of adults aged less than 65 years, 6 per cent of men and 12 per cent of women had a BMI below 20[6]. Low body mass in old age is associated with increased risk of morbidity and mortality[39]. A major hazard of being underweight is osteoporosis and tendency to fracture. Acute medical admissions and geriatric in-patients in Nottingham had lower body mass compared to the local normal values[34]. The vulnerability of elderly underweight people during intercurrent disease is likely to be greater because they lack metabolic resources needed at times of stress. Elderly people who are very thin may, for a long time, have been consuming a diet with multiple nutrient inadequacies in addition to energy deficit (para 4.5.1).

5.5.2   In the USA, the first National Health and Nutrition Examination included 2,777 white people aged 65-74 years old (1,314 men, 1,463 women) who were examined between 1971-75 and then again between 1982-84. The relationship of body mass to mortality was U-shaped with the lowest mortalities in the group of men with body mass index at the 60 to 84th percentiles and at the 40 to 59th percentiles for women. An increased risk of mortality was also observed in the black populations who were at the two ends of the range of percentiles for body mass index. Among older women, hip fracture was associated with extreme thinness[36].

Table 5.2: *Body mass index and energy intakes in elderly people 1972/73*[5]

Age 65–74 years

		Body Mass Index						
		< 20.0		20.0–25.0		25.1–30.0		30.1–40.0
	sex							
mean weight (kg)	M	52.7	(8)	65.6	(55)	75.8	(46)	89.9 (10)
	F	45.4	(8)	56.8	(38)	65.7	(26)	78.4 (13)
mean height (cm)	M	168	(8)	169	(55)	169	(46)	168 (10)
	F	157	(8)	157	(38)	155	(26)	156 (13)
mean energy intake (kcal)	M	2226	(8)	2413	(54)	2299	(46)	2713 (10)
	F	1718	(8)	1818	(36)	1808	(26)	1563 (13)

Age 75 years +

		< 20.0		20.0–25.0		25.1–30.0		30.1–40.0
	sex							
mean weight (kg)	M	53.8	(10)	62.8	(52)	73.3	(31)	85.3 (6)
	F	43.6	(10)	53.1	(34)	62.8	(20)	71.2 (7)
mean height (cm)	M	170	(10)	166	(52)	166	(31)	166 (6)
	F	153	(10)	153	(34)	153	(20)	150 (7)
mean energy intake (kcal)	M	2074	(10)	2118	(52)	2258	(31)	2149 (6)
	F	1505	(10)	1551	(34)	1617	(20)	1558 (7)

Figures in brackets are number of subjects in a cell

Total subjects: 65–74 years   M 119
                           F   85
        > 75 years   M   99
                           F   71

Table provided by Professor D J P Barker: Medical Research Council Clinical Epidemiology Unit, Southampton

5.5.3   There are public health benefits from avoiding underweight in elderly people. In accordance with usual clinical practices, progressive loss in weight should be taken as a signal for further investigations. When weight loss has occurred in an individual gradually over a long time it may be overlooked and health professionals and the general public need to be aware of the associated increased risks of morbidity and mortality.

5.6   Recommendations

1.   Further research should validate the best anthropometric methods for field work with elderly people.

2.   Demispan measurements should be extended to all nutritional surveys of elderly people and some of younger adults in order to assess its relationship to other measures of skeletal size and to parameters of health.

3.   The prognostic significance of body mass index and other anthropometric measures in a British population of elderly people should be clarified.

4.   Steps should be taken to increase the awareness by health professionals of the importance of both underweight and overweight in elderly people.

6. Nutrients: Carbohydrates and protein

6.1 Carbohydrate

6.1.1 *Dietary Sugars* Simple dietary sugars include monosaccharides, predominantly glucose and fructose, and disaccharides, predominantly sucrose and lactose. The major simple sugar consumed is sucrose. Between 10 and 20 per cent of food energy is presently obtained from simple sugars by the population as a whole, and elderly people may be closer to the upper end of this range because expenditure on sugar and preserves is greater in households with older housewives than in those with younger housewives[40]. In 1972/3, 12 per cent of food energy intake by elderly people was found to be derived from "added sugars" defined as sugars added to the foods during manufacture or processing in the kitchen or at table[5].

6.1.2 *Sugars and dental caries* Dental caries is related to the frequency and amount of intake of simple sugars. The COMA Panel on Dietary Sugars[41] defined the group of simple sugars associated with caries as "non-milk extrinsic sugars" which excludes lactose in milk and milk products and includes recipe sugars as added to composite dishes, soft drinks and confectionery, and table sugars added to a dish to the choice of the consumer, as well as sugars in fruit juices and honey. Based on a consideration of dental health, the Panel recommended that the intake of non-milk extrinsic sugars should be reduced. The COMA Panel on DRV recommended that for the populations as a whole an average of 10 per cent of food energy should come from this source. An upper limit for any individual of about 30 per cent of total food energy derived from non-milk extrinsic sugars has been advised under all circumstances, even for the edentulous, because intakes at this level or greater have been associated with adverse metabolic responses[41].

6.1.3 *Sugars and elderly people* The majority of elderly people will benefit from dietary modifications in line with these recommendations. A reduction in sugar intakes is especially important given the probability of higher than average consumption by elderly people (para 6.1.1). There has been a satisfactory trend to an increasing rate of retaining own teeth and this should not be reversed[42] (Table 6). Other factors which argue that young and old should be treated alike in making recommendations about the level of consumption of simple sugars, especially non-milk extrinsic sugars, include:

—the importance for elderly people of consuming a varied diet, including foods which are rich, on an energy basis, in vitamins and minerals (section 4.5). If large amounts of foods rich in simple sugars are consumed, appetite for a more varied and nutrient rich diet may be blunted;

23

—the increased liability of abnormal metabolic responses to a sucrose load in elderly people, especially the overweight and obese;

—the importance of retaining teeth to enable satisfactory chewing whether assisted with partial dentures, or not[43].

Table 6: *Proportion of edentulous people in Britain (per cent)*[42]

Year	Age (years)	Proportion edentulous (per cent)
1968	65–74	79
1978	65–74	74
1988	65–74	57
	65–69	49
	70–74	67
	75–79	75
	80 +	86

6.1.4 There may, however, be individual circumstances where appropriate intakes of simple sugars may be higher than the recommendations for the elderly population as a whole. Very elderly people, especially during episodes of ill health, may find difficulty in consuming sufficient dietary energy given that alternative energy sources such as fat may be less desirable or starchy foods may be difficult to consume. Sugar not only contains energy itself but may also help to increase the palatability to sick people and so encourage more food to be eaten.

6.1.5 *Complex Carbohydrates* The polysaccharides are chains of simple sugars. Dietary polysaccharides are divided into two main groups: starches which are alpha-glucan polysaccharides and may be long chain or branched, and non-starch polysaccharides described in para 6.1.7[1].

6.1.6 *Starches* In the 1972/3 nutritional survey of elderly people, 24 per cent of food energy was derived from bread and 8 per cent from potatoes with further contributions from other foods such as cakes and biscuits[5]. Starch provided 24 per cent of energy in the 1986/7 Dietary and Nutritional Survey of British Adults[6]. The COMA DRV Panel recommended that starches and intrinsic and milk sugars should contribute an overall 37 per cent of the total dietary energy for the population[1]. There are no recent data on the dietary intakes of these nutrients in an elderly population, but it is likely that this group, in common with all segments of the population, would benefit from an increased intake of starchy foods in the diet.

6.1.7 *Non-starch polysaccharides* (NSP) It has been difficult to assess claims for the therapeutic or preventive benefits of "dietary fibre" because it cannot be defined or measured precisely. Furthermore, "dietary fibre" intakes are often associated with intakes of other nutrients and it is difficult to isolate and examine independently the effects of varying levels of "fibre" intakes. The term non-starch polysaccharides comprise the major proportion of what is conventionally called "dietary fibre" but can be defined and measured

24

precisely. NSP include all the carbohydrates of the plant cell wall which are not digested and absorbed in the small intestine.

6.1.8 NSP are important in preventing constipation[44]. They increase stool weight and reduce bowel transit time and this effect is shared by certain forms of starch (resistant starch). Constipation is a common symptom which impairs the quality of life in about 20 per cent of elderly people[45]. For this reason, the recommendation from the COMA Panel on DRV, that NSP intakes should be increased by 50 per cent on average, from 12 g to 18 g per day, are applicable. Wholegrain cereals, pulses and some vegetables and fruit are high in NSP and these foods are recommended in particular because they are also valuable sources of several other nutrients. NSP may also be important in protecting against the development of diverticular disease and large bowel cancer. Because of its physical properties NSP may also moderate glucose and insulin metabolism and some may help to reduce blood cholesterol, but the doses required, and the degree to which these effects are independent of other dietary changes, are not yet clear.

6.1.9 Most elderly people enjoy foods high in NSP but a few who are edentulous, may have difficulty in chewing several of the foods which are rich in NSP. A few experience gaseous distension and discomfort partly due to fermentation of NSP in the large bowel. Raw bran contains phytate which binds to divalent mineral cations and reduces the availability of calcium, iron, copper and zinc. Excess intakes of food high in phytates, particularly unprocessed wheat bran or bran enriched products, should be avoided.

6.2 Protein

6.2.1 Total body protein contained in lean body mass falls with age, but there is great individual variation in the rate of decline (para 4.3). Protein synthesis[46], turnover[47] and breakdown[48] all decrease with advancing age. Protein utilisation and the homeostatic mechanisms which control appropriate increases in albumin synthesis with adequate dietary protein intake[49] may be less efficient in elderly people[7]. Furthermore, conditions of ill health, trauma, sepsis and immobilisation may upset the equilibrium between protein synthesis and degradation[48,50,51,52]. Adequate energy intake exerts a protein-sparing effect. It is important that elderly people maintain an adequate energy intake, especially during episodes of ill health when energy requirements may rise, in order to minimise protein loss.

6.2.2 The UK Reference Nutrient Intakes (RNI) for protein for the population aged 50 years or over are 46.5 g/d for women and 53.3g/d for men[1]. These values are in accord with the FAO/WHO/UNU daily recommendation of not less than 0.75 g good quality protein/kg body weight/d[7]. A recent study in Southampton[22] found healthy elderly subjects living at home and eating a self-selected diet, to be in metabolic equilibrium for protein on a mean daily intake of 69 g for men and 60 g for women, equivalent to 0.97 g mixed protein/ kg body weight/d. Metabolic equilibrium for protein in elderly subjects has been observed with daily intakes from 0.59 g to 0.80 g/kg body weight[21,53] although others have found 0.80 g/d insufficient[49]. Conditions varied between these studies and not all of the subjects were healthy.

6.2.3 The average protein intakes recorded in 1986/7 in adults aged 16 to 64 years were well in excess of RNI values and there was a trend to increasing intakes with age[6]. However, in the presence of disease the coincidence of low intake, inefficient homeostasis and possible attendant anabolic demands, may mean that a higher protein intake is necessary. Further research into the complex hormonal and non-hormonal mechanisms which control protein synthesis and degradation in health and disease, with particular reference to the vulnerable hospitalised elderly person, will be needed to formulate recommendations for these circumstances.

6.3 Recommendations

1. For the majority of elderly people, the same recommendations concerning the dietary intake of non-milk extrinsic sugars apply as for the younger adult population.

2. Intakes of NSP comparable to those recommended for the general population are advised for most elderly people. Foods with high phytate content, especially raw bran, should be avoided or used sparingly.

3. Further research should be done to determine, with more precision, the protein requirements of elderly people.

7. Nutrients: Vitamins

7.1 Vitamin A (retinol)

7.1.1 Vitamin A is needed for the maintenance of immune function, normal and night vision, and for the maintenance and repair of epithelial tissues. It can be obtained from animal sources in the diet as retinol, or from dietary carotenoids, such as beta-carotene. Overall one microgram of retinol is taken to be equivalent to 6 micrograms of dietary carotene. Carotenes, in addition to their effect as pro-vitamin A, have antioxidant properties, which it has been proposed may have some action in protecting against certain epithelial cancers, although evidence for this effect is far from conclusive[54].

7.1.2 The Dietary and Nutritional Survey of British Adults gave assurance that in 1986/7 the average vitamin A intake of adults aged less than 65 years was adequate[6]. The range of retinol equivalent intakes was wide and skewed and median intake values were all lower than the averages, although still adequate (Table 7). No cases of inadequate serum retinol concentration were found. It would be reasonable to extrapolate these findings to the British population of elderly people because there was a trend with increasing age towards higher intakes in both men and women. However, low intakes of vitamin A in individual elderly people have been reported in other countries and are probably due to personal dietary preferences[55]. The range of foods which are rich in retinol are limited to the animal products liver, egg yolk, milk fat, butter and cheese for retinol, and to yellow and orange vegetables, particularly carrots for carotenes. In the UK, yellow fats such as margarines are statutorily fortified with both vitamins A and D, and other fat spreads are fortified voluntarily by the manufacturers. The fortification of all yellow fats, except butter, is endorsed by the Working Group because it ensures an alternative source which continues to be consumed widely by elderly people in the UK[56].

Table 7: *Average daily intakes from food sources of retinol equivalents* * *(μg) by age and sex 1986/7*[6]

	Age (years)				All ages
	16–24	25–34	35–49	50–64	16–64
MEN					
Mean value	1164	1552	1759	1897	1628
Median value	786	965	1084	1132	1012
WOMEN					
Mean value	1051	1234	1531	1655	1413
Median value	633	719	884	951	810

*excludes any contribution from food supplements

27

7.2 Thiamin

7.2.1 In 1972/3 the average daily thiamin intake for elderly men was 1.0 mg and for women 0.8 mg[5]. Double this value was observed in the 1986/7 Dietary and Nutritional Survey of British Adults aged 16–64 years (2.0 mg/d in men; 1.6 mg/d in women)[6]. Information is lacking about whether the thiamin intakes of healthy elderly people have risen since 1972. Institutionalized elderly people probably have generally adequate intakes of thiamin although, since thiamin intakes are closely linked to the levels of energy intake, if the overall amount of food intake declines, thiamin intakes may not be adequate[57,58,59]. The methodology for assessing biochemical adequacy is limited. Drug-nutrient interactions and nutrient-nutrient interactions, especially with other B group vitamins[60] may partly explain why there is no simple relationship between level of thiamin intake and biochemical status. It has been suggested that thiamin deficiency is a factor in the development of confusional states[61]. Further research on thiamin status in vulnerable elderly subjects should pay particular regard to identifying the clinical features of early thiamin deficiency.

7.3 Riboflavin

7.3.1 Riboflavin is available from several food sources of which the chief is milk. There was no evidence of dietary intake levels below the RNI in either of the surveys of free living elderly or of younger adult populations[5,6]. However, a more recent dietary survey found that institutionalised elderly people are at risk of low intakes[58]. Furthermore, biochemical riboflavin deficiency was found in 30 per cent of the elderly subjects examined in 1972/3 (defined as erythrocyte glutathione reductase activation coefficient above 1.3) and this has been confirmed in other studies[57,62]. The relationship between nutrient intake and biochemical status is complex and non-dietary factors may have a substantial influence, especially in elderly people[63].

7.4 Vitamin B_{12}

7.4.1 Vitamin B_{12} (cyanocobalamin) is a constituent of the coenzymes involved in the conversion of the folates in the diet to active metabolites of folic acid[64]. Deficiency of either vitamin B_{12} or folate leads to megaloblastic anaemia. Vitamin B_{12} deficiency anaemia is usually caused by a failure of absorption and it is less commonly due to dietary deficiency. For absorption to occur, vitamin B_{12} must bind with "intrinsic factor" which is secreted by the stomach. If "intrinsic factor" ceases to be produced, as in pernicious anaemia, or as a result of gastrectomy or severe gastric atrophy, vitamin B_{12} cannot be absorbed. Absorption occurs in the terminal ileum, and if this segment of the gastro-intestinal tract is diseased, for example in Crohn's disease, the bound vitamin may fail to be absorbed. Vitamin B_{12} is present only in animal products. Except in very strict vegetarians, especially vegans, vitamin B_{12} deficiency anaemia is not usually caused by dietary deficiency although it has been suggested that, because of the high prevalence in elderly people of disorders which hinder absorption, higher dietary intakes may be beneficial[65].

7.4.2 There is some doubt whether serum vitamin B_{12} levels fall with age and, if so, whether it is due to decreased absorption or intake or both. A proportion of over 70 year olds have hypochlorhydria/achlorhydria and some of these may have impaired vitamin B_{12} absorption. No correlation was found between age and vitamin B_{12} absorption in a study of free living elderly people aged 60 to 90 years[66]. In 1972/3 the DHSS survey of elderly people found 17.9 per cent of the study group had serum vitamin B_{12} levels of 100–200 pg/ml (classified as "borderline") and 2.5 per cent had serum levels of less than 100 pg/ml (classified as "subnormal")[5]. The majority of studies reporting a fall in serum B_{12} levels have examined hospital populations, whereas those reporting no fall have examined elderly populations which are more broadly representative[67].

7.4.3   Replacement therapy for elderly individuals with low serum vitamin B_{12} levels but with no haematological abnormalities has been examined[68]. Thirty-nine non anaemic elderly subjects with serum vitamin B_{12} below 150 pg/ml showed no improvement in general wellbeing or in psychiatric state following 6 injections of vitamin B_{12}. In another study, when individuals with normal haematology but low serum vitamin B_{12} levels were followed up for ten years, blood indices remained normal without vitamin B_{12} therapy[69]. Nevertheless, the question of whether apathy, depression or mild cognitive impairment might be due to vitamin B_{12} deficiency remains unresolved and is an important area for clarification.

7.5   Folate

7.5.1   Folate deficiency leads to megaloblastic anaemia and macrocytosis. Iron deficiency can inhibit macrocytosis and hence mask this important sign of folate or vitamin B_{12} deficiency. Peripheral neuropathy sometimes occurs in people with deficiency of folate. A small number of cases of reversible severe dementia has been reported in association with folate deficiency[70]. Further work, using modern techniques, needs to be done to examine whether depression and mild cognitive impairment might follow folate deficiency.

7.5.2   The DHSS survey of elderly people in 1972/3 found 22 per cent of the group had borderline red cell folate levels and 5.4 per cent had subnormal values[5]. There was no evidence of clinical disorder due to folate deficiency in those found to have these low values, either in the 1972/3 DHSS study or in a large community study in South Wales[71]. In studies of healthy subjects aged over 75 years, slightly lower mean values were obtained than in younger individuals although they still lay within the normal adult range[72,73]. Many studies have shown that mean blood folate levels are lower in geriatric hospital patients than in the free living elderly population[74].

7.5.3   Prime sources of dietary folate are vegetables, liver and kidney. Folate is destroyed by prolonged cooking. Thus a "tea and toast" type of diet of some elderly people, and a tendency to overcook food, particularly in institutions, may contribute to dietary deficiency. Elderly people may also be at increased risk of folate deficiency because of small bowel disorders such as coeliac disease and bacterial overgrowth, which may interfere with absorption and which are not uncommon at this age.

7.6 Vitamin C

7.6.1 The RNI for vitamin C for adults is 40 mg/d and there is no evidence that this needs to be higher for elderly populations[1]. Fruit and vegetables provide vitamin C and these foods are the preferred sources because they contribute to the intakes of several other nutrients. Fortified drinks and vitamin C supplements may also be used to ensure adequate intakes especially for frail people with poor appetites. In 1972/3 the DHSS survey of elderly people recorded intakes of vitamin C which were below 40 mg/d for more than 50 per cent of both male and female groups and which were especially low in Scotland[5]. Although the 1986/7 Dietary and Nutritional Survey of British Adults aged 16 to 64 years reported mean levels of intake of vitamin C some 50 per cent higher than those recorded in 1972/3[6], it cannot be assumed that the vitamin C intakes in elderly people have also increased. Elderly people may have difficulties with preparing, peeling and chewing fruit and vegetables. Because of the rapid oxidation of vitamin C, especially over time and with heating, the vitamin C content of food may be depleted by the time it is consumed. "Meals on wheels" may lose up to 90 per cent of their vitamin C content by the time of delivery for this reason[75]. Those dependent on institutional catering may also be at particular risk of low intake[76].

7.6.2 Vitamin C deficiency which causes scurvy is only occasionally seen and these cases are generally associated with alcoholism or clinical disorders such as dementia. The role of vitamin C in connective tissue growth and wound healing is well recognised. Daily supplements of 1g vitamin C given to elderly institutionalised patients were associated with health improvements when compared to a placebo treated group[77]. There is no good evidence for the claim that supplements of vitamin C, at doses hundreds of times those needed to cure scurvy, are associated with better healing of pressure sores and leg ulcers.

7.6.3 Vitamin C is an important water soluble anti-oxidant and this effect in protecting against free radical-mediated oxidative tissue damage may have very wide implications in disease prevention. Specific disease processes, such as senile macular degeneration and cataract[78], as well as disorders of immune response (para 7.7.1), vascular disorders (para 9.3.1) and cancer (para 11.4) have been linked to oxidative damage mediated by free radicals. These observations underline the need for further examination for good biochemical indices of status, and of the consequences of chronic marginal vitamin C deficiency in elderly people.

7.7 Vitamin E

7.7.1 Vitamin E is an important lipid-soluble antioxidant. Normal immune function is influenced by vitamin E possibly through its effect on decreasing free radical formation (para 11.4) or by inhibiting prostaglandin synthesis or by other pathways as yet undetermined. A decline in immune responses with age is well established and this may be one of the determinants reducing longevity[79]. Clinical studies have not demonstrated an enhancement of the immune response as a result of increasing dietary vitamin E intake but definitive longitudinal studies have not been done[80]. There is some evidence from cross

30

country and clinical studies on younger adults that vitamin E may protect against atherosclerosis possibly by preventing lipid peroxidation and the liberation of damaging free radicals (para 9.3.1).

7.7.2   No EAR or RNI were set for vitamin E by the COMA Panel[1]. Dietary vitamin E requirements are largely determined by the polyunsaturated fatty acid (PUFA) content of the diet. Fortunately, foods naturally rich in these fats also generally contain vitamin E. Fats rich in PUFA, if taken as supplements, should also contain adequate amounts of vitamin E.

7.8   **Fruit and vegetables**   There are several reasons why an increased consumption of fruit and vegetables is desirable in the national diet. They contribute non-starch polysaccharides (para 6.1.8) and they are rich sources of vitamins and minerals. Several of these micronutrients have antioxidant properties and they may have a role in protecting against free oxidative radicals (para 11.4) which, it has been suggested, are concerned with the genesis of heart disease and other disorders (paras 7.6.3, 7.7.1, 8.5, 9.3.1). Any increased potassium intake which results from eating more fruit and vegetables is unlikely to cause adverse side effects and there may be a benefit from reduction in blood pressure.

7.9   **Recommendations**

1.   The statutory fortification of yellow fats other than butter with vitamin A and D should continue and manufacturers are encouraged to fortify other fat spreads voluntarily.

2.   The micronutrient intakes of elderly people in the UK need to be determined.

3.   The micronutrient requirements of the elderly population need to be determined more accurately.

4.   The clinical features of deficiency of vitamins from the B group especially thiamin, vitamin B_{12} and folate need to be investigated.

5.   Better biochemical indices of vitamin C status need to be developed.

6.   Elderly people should be encouraged to increase their dietary intakes of vitamin C.

7.   Adequate intakes of vitamin C need to be ensured for elderly people who are dependent on institutional catering.

8.   Elderly people, in common with those of all ages, should be advised to eat more fresh vegetables, fruit, and whole grain cereals.

8. Nutrients: Minerals

8.1 Magnesium

8.1.1 The RNI for magnesium is 12.3 μmol (300 mg)/d for men, 10.9 μmol (270 mg)/d for women; metabolic equilibrium was observed with intakes similar to this in 24 free living elderly people[22]. Potential causes of magnesium deficiency, such as low dietary intake and the use of diuretic therapy are more likely to occur in elderly people especially those who are ill. Further research is required to assess magnesium status in ill elderly people, particularly those with cardiac failure because cardiac arrhythmias may be potentiated by magnesium deficiency especially in the presence of other electrolyte imbalances.

8.2 Iron

8.2.1 Iron is essential for the synthesis of haemoglobin and for iron-containing enzymes and co-factors concerned with metabolic processes[81]. Average involuntary iron losses have been calculated as 11 μmol (0.61 mg)/d for elderly men and 11.5 μmol (0.64 mg)/d for elderly women, compared with 17 μmol (0.95 mg)/d for men and 22 μmol (1.24 mg)/d for women under 50 years of age[82]. Thus elderly people may have lower iron requirements to maintain an adequate iron status than when they were younger, and this applies particularly to women who no longer require iron to replace menstrual losses.

8.2.2 The assessment of iron status is not simple. Late manifestations of iron deficiency are a fall in blood haemoglobin and microcytosis, but neither is specific. Low serum ferritin more reliably indicates iron deficiency but high levels may be increased in inflammatory states or liver disease or other chronic disorders which tend to be more common in elderly people and do not necessarily imply good iron stores.

8.2.3 The efficiency of iron absorption depends on its form in the diet, the composition of the diet as a whole, the iron status of the individual, as well as the presence of general disorders such as infection or inflammatory states. Elderly people with iron deficiency can increase their iron absorption to the same extent as younger adults[83]. However, because of the higher prevalence in elderly people of disorders which interfere with efficient iron absorption, such as atrophic gastritis and post-gastrectomy syndromes, a proportion of the elderly population have reduced dietary availability of iron[81,84]. Blood loss associated with hiatus hernia, peptic ulcer, diverticular disease, haemorrhoids and cancer as well as with non-steroidal anti-inflammatory drug use, is more likely in elderly people. It is important to exclude other pathology as a cause of anaemia before assuming that it is due to a nutritional deficiency.

8.2.4 The COMA Panel on DRV recommended a RNI for iron of 160 μmol (8.7 mg)/d as adequate to meet the needs of the population of elderly men and women[1]. This value is based on an assumption that iron absorption from a diverse diet is no more than 15 per cent; hence the apparently high RNI when compared with the daily involuntary losses of iron described above. Even in diets which are providing iron intakes at or above the RNI, it is valuable to include foods containing haem-iron which is readily bioavailable, especially meat, preferably red meat or offal. Reducing agents in the diet, such as vitamin C, assist iron absorption. Some dietary components including phytates in bran, tannin in tea, or even other minerals such as copper and zinc, may interfere with iron absorption. Elderly individuals with high iron absorption may gradually accumulate iron in the body[81].

8.2.5   The British surveys of elderly people in 1972/3[5] and of adults aged 16 to 64 years in 1986/7[6] showed that a greater proportion of elderly than younger men had haemoglobin below a defined level. Women were more likely to have low haemoglobin levels at younger than at older ages (Table 8). In a detailed study of housebound and hospitalized elderly patients, the dietary iron intakes were lower than the intakes of a group of free living elderly people. However, when expressed in relation to caloric intake, the iron densities of the diets were similar for hospitalized and free living subjects[85]. This finding confirms the importance of maintaining an adequate food intake if micronutrient needs are to be met from a normal diet.

Table 8: *Proportion of British population with low haemoglobin (Hb) in DHSS diet and nutrition surveys*

Year of survey and age group	Men		Women	
	Total subjects	Proportion with low Hb*	Total subjects	Proportion with low Hb*
1972/3[5] aged > 68 years	166	17%	194	9%
1986/7[6] 16–64 years	846	2%	856	20%
50–64 years	231	2%	232	13%

*Definitions: 1972/3 (men Hb < 13 g/dl); (women Hb < 12 g/dl); 1986/7 (both sexes Hb < 12.5 g/dl)

8.3   Zinc

8.3.1   In the UK, healthy elderly people living at home and eating a self-selected diet were in metabolic balance for zinc on a mean daily intake of 137 μmol (9 mg) with leucocyte zinc levels comparable to healthy young people[22]. Institutionalised elderly subjects are at increased risk of zinc deficiency[86,87]. The beneficial effect of zinc to promote the healing of damaged tissues, especially skin, has been confirmed, but only in subjects who are zinc deficient[88]. Zinc deficiency adversely affects cellular immunity at all ages[89,90]. However, pharmacological doses of zinc may also impair cellular immunity[88] and may cause other adverse side effects[91,92].

8.4 Copper

8.4.1 Healthy elderly subjects in the UK were in metabolic balance for copper on a mean daily intake of 18.7 μmol (1.2 mg)[86]. Hospitalised elderly people had mean daily copper intakes of 13.2 μmol (0.8 mg) and their leucocyte copper levels (which may be a useful index of status) were very much lower compared to healthy elderly subjects studied by the same methods[86]. No clinical consequences have yet been identified in elderly people with this lower intake although animal studies suggest that catecholamine metabolism might be impaired[93]. Dietary copper requirements may be increased if the diet contains large amounts of raw bran or other foods containing phytate which binds to copper in an unabsorbable complex[94] (Para 6.1.9).

8.5 Selenium

8.5.1 Selenium occurs in cereals, fish and meat. Selenium levels in cereals are dependent on the selenium content of the soil where they have been grown so the selenium content of cereal foods varies. In the UK the diet provides adequate amounts. Both healthy and housebound elderly subjects have been observed to be in positive selenium balance on self selected diets[22]. Selenium supplements are not needed in the UK and should be avoided because high intakes are toxic; the maximum safe daily intake from all sources should not exceed 0.08 μmol (6 μg)/kg[1]. Low serum selenium levels are reported to be predictive of a wide variety of cancers[95,96]. The relationship between selenium status and the development of cancers has been the subject of intense study (para 11.4).

8.6 Recommendations

1. There should be further research to assess magnesium status in ill elderly people, particularly those with cardiac failure.

2. The iron status of elderly people in this country should be determined.

3. Clinical and biochemical markers of both zinc and copper status need to be defined more precisely.

9. Nutrition and vascular disease in later life

9.1 The main known environmental risk factors for cardiovascular disease are smoking and plasma lipid concentrations which are dominant for coronary heart disease (CHD), and high blood pressure which is dominant for risk of stroke. Dietary factors influence both plasma lipids and blood pressure. The Government recently set national targets for a health strategy which looks to a continuing improvement in the health of the nation[97]. Coronary heart disease and stroke were key areas for primary prevention and the relevant targets are:

— To reduce death rates for both CHD and stroke in people under 65 years by at least 40 per cent by the year 2000 (from 58 per 100,000 population in 1990 to no more than 35 per 100,000 for CHD, and from 12.5 per 100,000 population in 1990 to no more than 7.5 per 100,000 for stroke).
— To reduce the death rate for CHD in people aged 65 to 74 years by at least 30 per cent by the year 2000 (from 899 per 100,000 population in 1990 to no more than 629 per 100,000).
— To reduce the death rate for stroke in people aged 65 to 74 years by at least 40 per cent by the year 2000 (from 265 per 100,000 population in 1990 to no more than 159 per 100,000).

9.2 Diet and plasma lipids

9.2.1 *Plasma cholesterol and risk of CHD* Circulating levels of total cholesterol and its subfractions are among the most powerful known predictors of CHD in national and international comparisons. Risk of CHD is positively correlated with total cholesterol and with low density lipoprotein cholesterol (LDL) levels, and negatively correlated with levels of high density lipoprotein cholesterol (HDL). Inherent in the early speculations about this relationship was the idea that cholesterol which has found its way into arterial plaques was essentially 'fixed' in place and that therefore subsequent manipulation of plasma cholesterol could not be an effective preventive measure. There are several reasons now for doubting this concept, among the most convincing being angiographic studies showing that under favourable conditions, coronary arterial plaques can regress and over quite short periods of time[98]. Moreover, interventive studies indicate that the reduction in CHD risk associated with plasma cholesterol reduction is correspondingly rapid in onset.

9.2.2 *Longitudinal studies* Early data from the Framingham study on the relationship between plasma cholesterol and CHD seemed only to apply up to the age of about 55 years[99], and it was postulated that elderly people would be unlikely to benefit from a reduction in cholesterol levels as much as those who were younger. Such assumptions may have led to the frequent exclusion of older subjects from interventive trials of manipulating plasma cholesterol levels to reduce risk of CHD. More recent data from studies in the USA have shown that, although the *relative* risk of CHD associated with plasma cholesterol declines with age, it remains a predictor of CHD at least up to the age of 70 years and almost certainly beyond[100]. Furthermore, because of the high baseline risk of CHD in this age group, the absolute risk attributed to plasma cholesterol is much greater than at younger ages. The recent emergence of plasma cholesterol as a risk factor for CHD among elderly population samples in the USA may result from the declining mortality from CHD in the USA, which, since the late 1960s, has allowed the survival of a cohort of elderly people susceptible to the adverse effects of high plasma cholesterol levels, who in previous decades would have died in middle age[101]. Although the fall in mortality from CHD in the UK has been less and of shorter duration than that seen in the USA, it indicates that the UK may be in the process of repeating the USA experience of CHD risk factor status. An 18 year follow-up of the Whitehall study has recently confirmed the predictive value of raised plasma cholesterol for risk of death from CHD for elderly people in the UK[102].

9.2.3 It is unlikely that definitive observational studies on CHD risk factors in elderly populations will emerge in the near future. The interactions of risk factors such as plasma cholesterol, cigarette smoking, high blood pressure and body weight, obscure individual relationships with CHD. The absolute risk of CHD increases steeply with age (Figure 9), and advice for all adults, including elderly people, to adopt a diet that moderates plasma cholesterol levels is prudent. In contrast, if drug control of plasma cholesterol in later life is to be assessed it should be the subject of randomised controlled trials in view of the greater potential for hazards of drug treatments.

9.2.4 *Plasma triglycerides and risk of CHD* Plasma triglycerides have also been identified as a risk factor for CHD in some, but not in all studies. Their evaluation as an independent factor is complex because high triglyceride levels tend to be associated with low HDL cholesterol levels and with obesity, raised blood pressure and insulin resistance, all of which are also associated with increased risk of CHD. There are insufficient grounds at present for recommending specific dietary manipulation of plasma triglycerides as a means of affecting risk of CHD except where the elevation is extreme.

9.3 Damage to the arterial wall and thrombosis

9.3.1 Atherosclerosis results from cellular change in the endothelial lining and a chronic thickening of the arterial wall with smooth muscle hyperplasia, fibrosis and accumulation of lipid including cholesterol. Recently, the mechanisms which initiate plaque formation have focused on the possible role of free radical mediated oxidative modification of LDL. LDL cholesterol may be predominantly taken into the arterial wall by macrophages with receptors specific for its oxidised form, while modified LDL is less likely to be deposited. This process may be moderated through the antioxidant action of certain micronutrients particularly vitamins E[103] and C, carotene and selenium (para 11.4).

Death rates for Coronary Heart Disease
by sex and age   England   1991

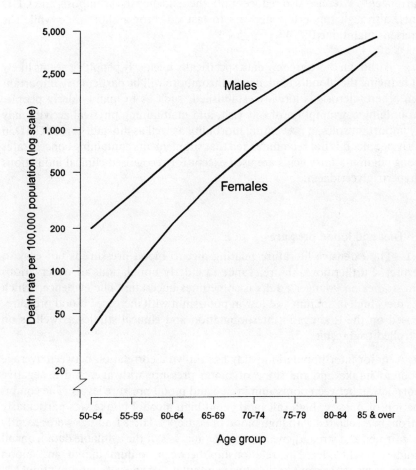

Source: OPCS (ICD 410:414)

Graphics by CHMU Jul 92

Figure 9

9.3.2 Luminal narrowing is associated not only with the atherosclerotic process, but also with repeated thrombosis over existing, often fissured, atherosclerotic plaques. In addition, the event leading to myocardial infarction is often thrombotic occlusion of a coronary artery, usually as a complication of rupture of an atherosclerotic plaque[104]. The possibility that dietary modification of thrombogenicity may affect the risk of CHD is supported by evidence of low CHD risk in populations with relatively high n-3 fatty acid intake (eg Eskimos), by clinical studies showing an effect on haemostasis of long-chain n-3 fatty acid supplementation, and by trials showing that dietary enrichment with n-3 fatty acids (either as oily fish or as a concentrate) in subjects who had already had one or more myocardial infarctions leads to a reduced rate of recurrence[105]. Exercise also reduces both the tendency to thrombosis and CHD events, although this effect appears to last only for a short time while the exercise is maintained[106,107].

9.3.3 Although there are few data specifically in elderly people, it seems likely that reducing the blood's tendency to thrombose will be particularly important when atherosclerosis is already established, such as in many elderly people. Encouraging consumption of oily fish, and maintaining physical activity may play important roles in preventing morbidity as well as mortality from CHD in elderly people. It is not recommended that supplements containing concentrates of long chain n-3 fatty acids are used except for recognised clinical indications eg hypertriglyceridaemia.

9.4 Diet and blood pressure

9.4.1 The extensive literature relating diet to blood pressure is not easy to interpret. Furthermore, the relevance to elderly populations of observations from studies on younger adults is sometimes uncertain. The evidence, which links diets high in sodium and low in potassium with increased blood pressure, is based on the findings in interpopulation and clinical studies as well as on controlled trial results.

a. A major inter-population study has shown a correlation between average sodium intake and the slope of blood pressure with age, and a negative correlation between potassium intake and blood pressure levels. The combination of obesity, high salt intake and high alcohol intake was particularly strongly associated with high blood pressure[108]. These findings were recently confirmed and strengthened by further analysis of the available data from all studies worldwide. The relationship between sodium intake and blood pressure was consistent both between populations and within populations[109].

b. Clinical studies in which manipulations of dietary sodium and potassium have brought about changes in blood pressure in human subjects provide further evidence[110,111]. Older people may be more responsive to reductions in sodium intake than those who are younger although this requires more critical study[110]. It has also been suggested that the chloride ion may independently be important in enhancing the effect of dietary sodium on blood pressure[112].

c. There is evidence that public health benefits in this respect are achievable. A controlled trial in Portugal has shown that a health education programme aimed at reducing high salt intake resulted in a reduction of the whole community blood pressure distribution sufficient to reduce mean values by 5 mm Hg over two years[113].

9.4.2 Overall reduction in salt intake seems likely to produce a long-term reduction in prevailing blood pressure levels and in particular, in the rate of increase of blood pressure with age. The UK RNI for adults for sodium is 70 mmol/d (equivalent to 4 g salt/d) which is the level to ensure adequacy in the population[1]. The World Health Organisation has recently suggested that 6g salt/d may be a reasonable upper population average for salt intake[44]. Current intakes by adults in the UK average about 9 g/d. Elderly people on very reduced salt diets may have difficulty in compensating for salt losses induced by severe sweating, vomiting or diarrhoea. These hazards are extremely unlikely from salt reductions which approach WHO recommendations. Therefore, with caution relating to special circumstances, the elderly population, in common with younger age groups, would be expected to benefit from a reduction in average salt intakes. If average blood pressure levels were lowered by dietary means the consequent need for pharmacological intervention would be reduced.

9.5 Recommendations

1. Elderly people should be encouraged to adopt diets which moderate their plasma cholesterol levels.

2. There should be encouragement of elderly people to consume oily fish and to maintain physical activity in order to reduce the risk of thrombosis.

3. The Working Group endorsed the WHO recommendation that 6 g/d sodium chloride would be a reasonable average intake for the elderly population in the UK, and recommends that the present average dietary salt intakes be reduced to meet this level.

10. Nutrition and bone health in elderly people

10.1 Osteoporosis

10.1.1 Osteoporosis is a disorder characterised by a reduction in bone mass associated with an increased rate of fracture particularly of vertebra, wrist and femoral neck. It is predominantly a condition of middle life and old age and it affects women more than men. There has been a steady increase in the number of admissions to hospital for hip fracture over the last three decades, due both to the demographic trend towards an ageing population and to an increase in the age-specific incidence of the fracture although this latter trend may now have ceased[114]. There were about 46,000 cases of this type of fracture in the UK in 1985 associated with considerable morbidity, mortality and economic costs[115].

10.1.2 Bone mass changes throughout life with a maximum (peak bone mass) achieved in young adulthood and bone loss after the fourth decade. The rates of decline vary between individuals but tend to be constant within each individual although there is a perimenopausal increase in the rate in women. Genetic, hormonal, mechanical and nutritional factors influence the attainment of peak bone mass, the onset of bone loss and the rate of bone loss. After the menopause there is a decline in oestrogen production which is associated with bone loss. Other factors associated with lower bone mass in adults include, low body weight, smoking, alcohol consumption, reduced physical activity, low calcium absorption and causes of secondary osteoporosis such as steroid therapy.

10.2 Calcium

10.2.1 The role of nutritional factors in the pathogenesis of osteoporosis remains unclear. There is some evidence that a dietary intake of calcium of less than 20 mmol (800 mg)/d during childhood and early adult life may be associated with a lower peak bone mass[116]. The relationships between bone mass and calcium balance at older ages must be set in the context of peak bone mass and its variability between individuals. Peak bone mass is generally an unknown confounding variable in examining the determinants of osteoporosis unless the follow-up extends for a very long time in studies begun in young adults. Metabolic balance studies may also be difficult to interpret because adaptation to a changed dietary intake may continue for several months, and it may take a long time to develop a steady state. During this time there is little relationship between calcium intakes and bone loss[117,118]. It is also likely that there is a genetic heterogeneity in ability to adapt to low calcium diets which will exert an influence on calcium status at all ages.

10.2.2 The limited available information in elderly people suggests that a dietary calcium intake of less than 500 mg/d in elderly people is associated with a lower cortical but not trabecular bone mass, although this may reflect an earlier effect of calcium intake during growth on peak bone mass rather than a subsequent effect on bone loss. Some studies have shown an apparent reduction in the incidence of femoral fractures with a dietary calcium intake above 20–25 mmol (800–1000 mg)/d[119,120] although this is by no means a universal observation[121,122]. Although high calcium intakes of 25 to 37.5 mmol(1 to 1.5 g)/d have been recommended[123] these are probably unnecessary and difficult to maintain on a normal diet. Where vitamin D activity is reduced the efficiency of calcium absorption from the gut declines[124,125] (para 10.3.1). Ensuring that elderly people are vitamin D replete appears to prevent the decline in calcium absorption and reduces the rate of cortical bone loss[124,126].

10.2.3 The RNI for adults and elderly people for calcium and phosphorus were set equimolar at 17.5 mmol/d (700 mg/d for calcium and 550 mg/d for phosphorus)[1]. The COMA Panel on DRV found no basis to recommend an increased intake of calcium or phosphorus in those aged 50 years or more so long as adequate vitamin D status was maintained. However, the Panel acknowledged that the data on which to base these recommendations were very limited. Dietary phosphorus intakes in both free living and housebound elderly people have been recorded well above the RNI[127].

10.2.4 In view of the uncertainty about the role of dietary calcium in the pathogenesis of osteoporosis, it is prudent that calcium intakes should not fall below current levels. Because there are few calcium rich foods, the potential for elderly people to have low dietary calcium intakes is very real. Major sources of calcium and phosphorus in the diet are milk and milk products. Households of elderly people generally consume more milk than other households although the intake has declined for all. Between 1975 to 1990 the mean total milk and cream consumed by elderly households declined from 5.57 pints to 4.31 pints per week[128]. The proportion of households buying milk from a milkman declined from 82 per cent in 1985 to 68 per cent in 1990[129]. Doorstep deliveries of milk are an accessible supply for elderly people and any reduction could lead to reduced milk consumption. In the UK white flour is fortified with calcium carbonate, and it, and products made from it, vegetables and hard water also contribute calcium in the diet.

10.3 Vitamin D

10.3.1 The predominant source of vitamin D in humans is from the skin through the exposure of the precursor 7-dehydrocholesterol to ultra-violet irradiation[130]. The diet provides smaller amounts of vitamin D, which are essential when cutaneous production is limited. Vitamin D itself has little biological activity, and is converted in the liver to 25 hydroxyvitamin D (25 OHD) which is the major circulating metabolite. This undergoes further hydroxylation in the kidneys to form the hormonally active metabolite of vitamin D, 1,25 dihydroxyvitamin D (1,25(OH)$_2$D). Vitamin D status may be compromised by malabsorption or gastric surgery. Anticonvulsant therapy or liver disease interferes with the efficient hepatic metabolism of vitamin D, and may add to the problems of maintaining adequate vitamin D status[131].

10.3.2 *Osteomalacia* The major clinical manifestation of vitamin D deficiency in adults is osteomalacia. This is a generalised bone disorder, characterised by an impairment of mineralisation which leads to the accumulation of unmineralised matrix or osteoid in the skeleton. The two commonly used markers of vitamin deficiency are low plasma 25 OHD concentration, and a histological diagnosis of osteomalacia. Plasma 25 OHD levels of 25–75 nmol/1 are taken as normal. In osteomalacia levels are usually below 10 nmol/1 and are associated with raised plasma parathyroid hormone concentrations[132]. Osteomalacia is essentially a histological diagnosis, so there is limited information on its prevalence. Two histological studies from Leeds suggest that 12–20 per cent of patients with femoral fracture have evidence of osteomalacia[133,134] although studies from London and Cardiff showed a much lower prevalence[121,135]. This may reflect a true geographical variation.

10.3.3 *Vitamin D and sunlight* Exposure to sunlight can be sufficient to ensure vitamin D adequacy. Even short periods of summer sunlight (15–30 minutes per day) with exposure of forearms, hands and face will lead to the production of adequate amounts[136]. However, because of the northerly latitude of the UK, ultraviolet light of the wavelength required for vitamin D production (290–315 nm) only reaches northern regions of the UK between May and September. The ultraviolet light of longer wavelength which penetrates in winter, may cause photodegradation of vitamin D[137].

10.3.4 If people become less mobile or housebound, it becomes increasingly difficult to obtain adequate vitamin D from the action of sunlight on the skin, especially in northern Britain[138]. Where possible, convenient seats in wind-sheltered spots may allow elderly people to enjoy the sunshine. Special glass which transmits the beneficial ultraviolet wavelengths is available, and may be installed in housing for elderly people. The benefit of deriving vitamin D through exposing skin to sunlight needs to be described in health education for elderly people. This is especially relevant where there is a cultural tradition of covering nearly all the body in clothes.

10.3.5 *Dietary intakes of vitamin D* It may be difficult to achieve a diet that, by itself, is adequate in vitamin D because the foods which are naturally rich in vitamin D are limited to fatty fish, eggs and liver. Butter contains smaller amounts. There has been a long standing requirement in the UK to fortify margarine with vitamins A and D. The COMA Working Group on the Fortification of Yellow Fats with Vitamins A and D has recommended that this practice should continue because it is a major contribution to vitamin D intakes in the UK especially for elderly people[56]. Several breakfast cereals are now fortified with vitamin D but the importance of this as a contribution to vitamin D intakes by elderly people is uncertain.

10.3.6 It has been estimated that the mean dietary intake of vitamin D is in the region of 2.0 μg/d[1], whilst an intake of 5–10 μg/d is required to ensure plasma

25 0HD concentrations above the level associated with osteomalacia in the absence of a contribution from cutaneous synthesis[139]. A recent study from USA has shown that dietary supplementation with vitamin D in winter leads to reduced seasonal bone loss in postmenopausal women[140]. The COMA Panel on DRV recommended that a vitamin D intake of 10 μg/d should meet the needs of virtually all people aged 65 years or above in this country[1]. Vitamin D supplementation should therefore be considered in those who are housebound or institutionalised, in a dose to provide a daily total of 10 μg/d, which may be given as a daily supplement or as 6 monthly or annual depot injections[141].

10.4 Fluoride A high fluoride intake in drinking water of 4–6 parts per million is associated with a higher bone mass[142,143]. A lower rate of vertebral and femoral fractures has also been claimed[142,144], although the reduction in fracture incidence is not a universal finding[143]. Sodium fluoride has also been used in the treatment of established osteoporosis, but whilst it increases trabecular bone mass by up to 35 per cent, this appears to be at the expense of cortical bone mass. Furthermore, sodium fluoride treatment does not reduce the incidence of vertebral crush fractures, and may increase the number of non-vertebral fractures[145].

10.5 Recommendations

1. Research is needed into the nutritional component to the attainment of peak bone mass.

2. Further studies are needed to determine optimal intakes of calcium for the elderly population.

3. The calcium intakes of elderly people in the UK should be monitored.

4. Doorstep deliveries of milk for elderly people should be maintained.

5. Research is needed on the clinical features of vitamin D deficiency.

6. All elderly people should be encouraged to expose some skin to sunlight regularly during the months May to September.

7. If adequate exposure to sunlight is not possible, vitamin D supplementation should be considered especially during the winter and early spring.

11. Nutrition and cancer

11.1 **Epidemiology** In the UK, 64 per cent of all new cancers occur in the 65 year and over age group[146]. Epidemiological studies provide most of the evidence for the dietary associations with the aetiology of cancer[147]. The range of cancers involved, and the multitude of variables which confound the assessment of the data, make precise relationships elusive at this stage but some general trends have emerged[44]. There is some evidence from cross country studies that, in the long term, high fat diets are associated with colon, breast and prostatic cancers. In these studies calories, dietary fat and obesity are all inter-related variables and their relative significance in the aetiology of cancer remains unclear[148]. As the basis of healthy dietary habits, elderly people should be advised to avoid long term high fat intakes because, among other benefits, lower fat intakes may help to reduce their risk of cancer. High consumption of fruit and vegetables have been inversely related to the risk of cancer. A prospective study of elderly people in Massachusetts demonstrated significant decreased risk of all cancers associated with increased consumption of carotenoid containing vegetables[149].

11.2 Free radicals and lipid peroxidation

11.2.1 A biological mechanism which may provide a theoretical basis for some of the associations between the development of cancer and nutritional status invokes the damaging oxidative effects on cells of oxygen-derived species such as hydrogen peroxide or free radicals such as hydroxyl or superoxide. These highly active species have the capacity to damage cellular components by oxidation at any site where they are produced. The extent of damage is dependent both on the activity and on the biological half life of the radical. Radicals produced intracellularly can damage DNA and lead to mutations.

11.2.2 Radicals are produced in the course of normal , oxidative metabolism, as a result of cytochrome P_{450} activity and as part of the respiratory burst of activated phagocytes in cell mediated immunity. To counteract the undesirable effects of the oxidative process, there are two main groups of natural antioxidants[150]: preventive substances such as carotenoids and riboflavin, which are mainly iron chelators or binding compounds, and radical scavengers which include superoxide dismutase, vitamins E and C, urate and beta-carotene. Selenium is essential for glutathione peroxidase which can metabolise lipid peroxides to harmless fatty acids. Although a number of the components involved in these reactions (substrates, catalysts, antioxidants) are derived from the diet, it is not established to what extent the dietary intakes of individual nutrients determines their activity. There is currently no single accepted method for determining overall antioxidant status *in vivo*.

11.3 **Diet and cancer** Within the tissues, the balance between free radical activity and antioxidant status is important for the maintenance of cellular integrity. The major dietary contributors to that balance are those vitamins and minerals which enhance antioxidant activity. These include beta-carotene (para 7.1.1) and possibly other carotenoids, vitamins (para 7.6.3) and E (para 7.7.1) and selenium (para 8.5). These nutrients occur particularly in fresh vegetables and fruit and cereals, which are foods whose consumption is already being encouraged in the UK as contributing to a healthy diet (see Chapter 7, recommendation 8). Although the precise nutrient relationships are unclear, a diet of vegetables and fruit is also likely to be high in complex carbohydrates and low in fat and energy, all of which have been associated with lower incidence of cancer. Such a diet can, therefore, be recommended with greater confidence than any individual component.

11.4 **Recommendations**

1. The relationships between the development of cancer and dietary energy and nutrients should continue to be investigated.

2. Methodologies should be developed for the determination of antioxidant status.

12. The impact of ill health on the nutrition of elderly people

12.1   Ill health frequently has an adverse effect on nutritional status especially in elderly people. For most, these effects are limited to the time of acute illness and the temporary nutritional disadvantage is overcome once their customary pattern of eating is resumed. If episodes of ill health occur repeatedly, nutritional status may decline step by step. The 1967/68 DHSS survey showed that elderly people who believed that they had a poorer health status than average tended to have lower energy intakes and lower body weights[4]. A study in 1986 showed that weight, body composition and dietary intakes were markedly different in samples of elderly people who were day patients or inpatients when compared with the free living elderly population (Table 12.1)[151]. A housebound group of people in Southampton, aged from 69 to 85 years, suffering from various chronic disorders although known hepatic, renal, gastro-intestinal diseases, malignancies and acute illnesses were excluded, had diets that were at greater risk of deficiencies of protein, zinc, copper, iron, selenium, calcium and phosphorus when compared with those of apparently healthy people of similar age[22]. The true prevalence of nutritional deficiencies

Table 12.1: *Nutritional status of elderly women in different clinical groups*[151]

Elderly female group	No.	Mean age (range) (yr)	Mean weight (kg)	Mean lean body mass (kg)	Mean total body fat (kg)	Mean energy intake (kcal/d)*	Mean protein intake g/d*
a) Active elderly women	57	73(69–78)	64	42	22	1,864	68
b) Day centre clients	75	81(65–94)	60	41	19	1,565	59
c) Geriatric day hospital patients	46	81(63–93)	55	39	16	—	—
d) Geriatric longstay patients	71	84(61–101)	48	35	13	1,541	52
e) Geriatric acute or chronic longstay patients	20	82(69–92)	48	35	13	1,269	46

*Nutrient intakes derived using differing methodologies:
a)   25 of total group kept 7 day weighed record
b)   17 of total group kept 7 day descriptive record
d & e) known food supplied less food wasted (all women).

may be underestimated because many studies in residential/nursing homes exclude ill or frail residents from their samples and it is these individuals who are likely to have particularly low energy and nutrient intakes.

12.2 Ill health and reduced food intake Studies of elderly people in hospitals and residential/nursing homes are in agreement that food intakes are less than those reported for free-living elderly people[152,153,154]. Long-stay geriatric inpatients studied in Southampton had energy intakes in 19 of 21 cases which were below $1.27 \times$ BMR and they consistently lost weight over a one year period[86]. Illness may cause reduced food intake for several reasons.

a. There may be impairment of appetite. The appreciation of both taste and flavour can be reduced substantially in elderly people and may be badly compromised both by illness and by many of the drugs commonly prescribed.

b. The sick may be unable to buy, prepare, and cook food for themselves. Those needing assistance with feeding are especially vulnerable.

c. Mental state is important. Elderly people who are confused cope poorly with preparing and eating food whilst those who are depressed may have anorexia.

d. Poor oral health and poor dentition may hinder an adequate dietary intake[43].

e. Gastrointestinal disease or drug therapy may cause nausea, vomiting, dysphagia, dyspepsia, steatorrhoea or diarrhoea which have a direct impact on food intake or absorption.

12.3 Altered physical activity in the sick

12.3.1 Activity generally falls during illness. In long term illness lean body mass declines, and hence BMR also may tend to fall. However, some illnesses may be associated with an increased muscle activity resulting from disease processes which gives rise to increased energy needs. Manifestations of illness, such as breathlessness, have a considerable energy cost although this has not been quantified in the elderly. Elderly Parkinson's disease sufferers had a 25 per cent increase in resting energy expenditure when compared with controls, which suggests that muscle rigidity and involuntary movements have a considerable energy cost[155]. Well elderly females have a higher energy cost for free walking compared to younger females (para 4.6.4), and more major disabilities which impair the mechanical efficiency of movement must increase the energy needs, although this appears not to have been studied in elderly people.

12.3.2 People suffering from dementia may be very active, they often eat poorly and a high proportion are very thin[156]. In a study of 18 elderly women (15 were very thin) in a chronic mental illness hospital, energy intakes (measured by 7 day weighed food intakes) and energy outputs (measured by the doubly labelled water technique) found none of the patients to be in significant energy imbalance[157]. This raises the possibilities either that negative energy balance may be episodic during periods of superimposed acute illnesses, or that the loss of lean body mass results in energy balance being achieved at a lower intake and expenditure.

12.4 Energy and nutrient cost of metabolic disturbances of illness The extra energy and nutrient costs of the metabolic changes associated with illness or disability are those most likely to go unrecognised. Many illnesses, infections, inflammatory states, trauma (including surgery), tissue necrosis or tumours, set in train metabolic changes which appear to have value in terms of host defence. These include fever, in which the basal metabolism rises by about 10 per cent for each degree centigrade of temperature elevation, although there is a considerable range of variation[158]. The acute-phase response remains fully active, even in advanced old age[159]. Acute-phase proteins are all synthesised in the liver, some in quite large amounts and this may impose a significant energy cost. In contrast, leucocytosis is often reduced or absent in old age. It is difficult to quantify these and other metabolic costs separately, but in one study, chest infection in elderly patients was accompanied by a 32.5 per cent rise in resting energy expenditure even though average rise in body temperature was only $1\,^\circ C$[160]. This suggests that the energy costs other than fever were of the order of 20 per cent of resting energy expenditure. Whilst metabolic changes have generally been studied in acute illness, they may persist in chronic illnesses. Rheumatoid arthritis for example leads to long-term activation of the acute-phase response indicating that there may be a continuing energy and nutrient penalty.

12.5 Nutritional status of elderly patients

12.5.1 In 1974, a single day survey in an American hospital of 131 surgical patients, including some with cancer, found that approximately 50 per cent were inadequately nourished[161]. Similar findings have been reported from this country[162]. Another study found that indices of nutritional abnormality were most frequent (50 per cent) in those patients who remained in hospital for more than a week after major surgery, and who were presumably more seriously ill, and that most of these abnormalities had gone unrecognised[163]. Medical patients in the same study also had a high risk of nutritional inadequacy and suffered caloric depletion, but had better protein status than the surgical patients. More recent studies continue to show that nutrient deficiencies are more common in hospitalized elderly people[58,153]. Poor nutritional status is a risk factor for morbidity and mortality. In a series of 304 admissions to a geriatric unit, weight, mid arm circumference, triceps skinfold thickness, albumin, retinol binding protein and plasma retinol were all significantly lower in patients who died[164]. Likewise, the predictive power of poor nutritional status for long term health problems is greater than that of age (para 5.5.1).

12.5.2 Improving the nutrition of elderly people in hospital or residential homes There are few reports of methods for improving food intake and nutritional status of elderly people living in residential or nursing homes. When the intakes in two nursing homes routinely serving three or five meals daily were compared, it was found that, except for energy for men in one home, either approach resulted in sufficient food intake, although in both homes food was refused. Most nutrients were consumed in slightly larger amounts in the home serving five meals, but these differences were not statistically significant[165]. Four factors have been found to be influential in optimising intake in patients with Alzheimer's disease, using skilled feeding techniques, selecting appropriate food consistency, providing adequate time, and capitalizing on the midday meal when cognitive abilities were at their peak[166]. This indicates that ensuring an adequate food intake for people living in institutions has implications both for clinical services and for administration.

12.5.3   Other attempts to improve nutritional status have focused on the use of supplements. When overnight tube feeding was used to supplement the dietary intakes of patients with fractured neck of femur[167], the sum of voluntary and supplemental intakes was greater than in the control group, and almost equal to that of a group of well-nourished patients. Furthermore, significant increases were found in weight, arm circumference and skinfold thickness in the supplemented group. However, a fall in serum albumin, prealbumin and transferrin, presumably as part of the acute-phase response to injury, was unaffected by tube feeding except for a more rapid return to normal of prealbumin in the very thin group receiving the supplement. Time to independent mobility was shortened by daily oral supplementation which was continued for a mean of 32 days. The supplemented patients continued to have a lower rate of complications 6 months later[168]. Benefits to nutritional status have been found using differing methods of supplementation, including milk based preparations[169] and a specially formulated liquid meal replacement[170]. Non-compliance with oral supplementation may be a problem. In a study of sip-feed supplementation out of 30 patients, 11 refused sip feeds altogether and none chose to consume large daily amounts[171].

12.5.4   Assessment of the nutritional status of elderly people admitted to hospital should be a routine aspect of history taking and physical examination. Formal nutritional therapy including supplements if necessary, should be instituted for undernourished elderly people during hospital admission especially following trauma or after surgery. In the longer term every encouragement should be for the patient to eat more solid food especially after going home.

12.6   Recommendations

1.   The impact of acute and chronic illness on the nutritional requirements of the elderly needs comprehensive study.

2.   Parameters of nutritional status with prognostic significance in ill elderly patients should be determined.

3.   Health professionals should be made aware of the impact of nutritional status on the development of and recovery from illness.

4.   Health professionals should be aware of the often inadequate food intake of elderly people in institutions.

5. Assessment of nutritional status should be a routine aspect of history taking and clinical examination when an elderly person is admitted to hospital.

6. Effective methods of ensuring adequate nutrition need to be developed and evaluated especially for elderly people in hospital or institutions.

13. References

1. Department of Health. *Dietary Reference Values for Food Energy and Nutrients for the United Kingdom*. London: HMSO, 1991. (Reports on health and social subjects; 41).

2. Department of Health and Social Security. *Interim Report on Vitamin D by the Panel on Child Nutrition—First Report by the Panel on Nutrition of the Elderly*. London: HMSO, 1970. (Reports on public health and medical subjects; 123).

3. Department of Health. *On the State of the Public Health: The Annual Report of the Chief Medical Officer of the Department of Health for the Year 1990*. London: HMSO, 1991.

4. Department of Health and Social Security. *A Nutrition Survey of the Elderly*. London: HMSO, 1972. (Reports on health and social subjects; 3).

5. Department of Health and Social Security. *Nutrition and Health in Old Age*. London: HMSO, 1979. (Report on health and social subjects; 16).

6. Gregory J, Foster K, Tyler H, Wiseman M. *The Dietary and Nutritional Survey of British Adults*. London: HMSO, 1990.

7. World Health Organization. *Energy and Protein Requirements. Report of a Joint FAO/WHO/UNU Expert Consultation*. Geneva: World Health Organization, 1985. (WHO Technical Report Series; 724).

8. Durnin JVGA. Energy intake, energy expenditure and body composition in the elderly. In: Chandra RK, ed. *Nutrition, Immunity and Illness in the Elderly*. New York: Pergamon Press, 1985; 19–33.

9. Fredrix EWHM, Soeters PB, Deerenberg IM, Kester ADM, von Meyenfeldt MF, Saris WHM. Resting and sleeping energy expenditure in the elderly. *Eur J Clin Nutr* 1990; **44**: 741–747.

10. Schoeller DA. Energy expenditure from doubly labelled water: some fundamental considerations in humans. *Am J Clin Nutr* 1983; **38**: 999–1005.

11. Coward WA. The $^2H_2$ ^{18}O technique: principles and practice. *Proc Nutr Soc* 1988; **47**: 209–218.

12. Schofield WN, Schofield C, James WPT. Basal metabolic rate—review and prediction. *Hum Nutr: Clin Nutr* 1985; **39C (Suppl)**: 1–96.

13. James WPT. Energy. In: Horwitz A et al, eds. *Nutrition in the Elderly*. Oxford: Oxford University Press, 1989; 49–64.

14. Knight I, Eldridge J. *The Heights and Weights of Adults in Great Britain*. London: HMSO, 1984.

15. Dallosso HM, Morgan K, Bassey EJ, Ebrahim SBJ, Fentem PH, Arie THD. Levels of customary physical activity among the old and the very old living at home. *J Epidemiol Community Health* 1988; **42**: 121–127.

16. Moreiras-Varela O, van Staveren WA, Amorim Cruz JA, Nes M, Lund-Larssen K. Intake of energy and nutrients. *Eur J Clin Nutr* 1991; **45, Suppl 3**: 105–119.

17. Lundgren BK, Steen B, Isaksson B. Dietary habits in 70 and 75-year old males and females. Longitudinal and cohort data from a population study. *Naringforskning* 1987; **31**: 53–56.

18. Durnin JVGA. Food intake and energy expenditure of elderly people. *Clin Geront* 1961; **4**: 128–133.

19. McGandy RB, Barrows CH, Spanias A, Meredith A, Stone JL, Norris AH. Nutrient intakes and energy expenditure in men of different ages. *J Geront* 1966; **21**: 581–587.

20. Borgstrom B, Norden A, Akesson B, Abdulla M, Jagerstad M. Nutrition and old age. Chemical analyses of what old people eat and their states of health during a 6 year follow-up. *Scand J Gastro-ent* 1979; **52** (suppl): 1–299.

21. Uauy R, Scrimshaw NS, Young VR. Human protein requirements: Nitrogen balance response to graded levels of egg protein in elderly men and women. *Am J Clin Nutr* 1978; **31**: 779–785.

22. Bunker VW, Clayton BE. Research Review: Studies in the nutrition of elderly people with particular reference to essential trace elements. *Age Ageing* 1989; **18**: 422–429.

23. Loenen HMJA, Eshuis H, Lowik MRH, Schouten EG, Hulshof KFAM, Odink J, Kok FJ. Serum uric acid correlates in elderly men and women with special reference to body composition and dietary intake (Dutch Nutrition Surveillance System). *J Clin Epidemiol* 1990; **43**: 1297–1303.

24. Voorrips LE, van Staveren WA, Hautvast JGAJ. Are physically active elderly women in a better nutritional condition than their sedentary peers? *Eur J Clin Nutr* 1991; **45**: 545–552.

25. Royal College of Physicians. *Medical aspects of exercise: benefits and risks*. London: Royal College of Physicians of London, 1991.

26. Office of Population, Censuses and Surveys. *General Household Survey 1986*. London: HMSO, 1989.

27. Patrick JM, Bassey EJ, Irving JM, Blecher A, Fentem PH. Objective measurements of customary physical activity in elderly men and women before and after retirement. *Quart J Exp Physiol* 1986; **71**: 47–58.

28. Bassey EJ, Terry AM. The oxygen cost of walking in the elderly. *J Physiol* 1986; **373**: 42P.

29. Bassey EJ, Terry AM. Blood lactate in relation to oxygen uptake during uphill treadmill walking in young and old women. *J Physiol* 1988; **396**: 104P.

30. Aniansson A, Grimby G, Rundgren A. Isometric and isokinetic quadriceps muscle strength in 70 year old men and women. *Scand J Rehabil Med* 1980; **12**: 161–168.

31. Fiatarone MA, Marks EC, Ryan ND, Meredith CN, Lipsitz LA, Evans WJ. High intensity strength training in nonagenarians. Effects on skeletal muscle. *J Am Med Assoc* 1990; **263**: 3029–3034.

32. Bassey EJ. Demispan as a measure of skeletal size. *Ann Hum Biol* 1986; **13**: 499–502.

33. Rolland-Cachera MF, Cole TJ, Sempe M, Tichet J, Rossignol C, Charraud A. Body Mass Index variations: Centiles from birth to 87 years. *Eur J Clin Nutr* 1991; **45**: 13–21.

34. Lehmann AB, Bassey EJ, Morgan K, Dallosso HM. Normal values for weight, skeletal size and body mass indices in 890 men and women aged over 65 years. *Clin Nutr* 1991; **10**: 18–22.

35. Burr ML, Phillips KM. Anthropometric norms in the elderly. *Br J Nutr* 1984; **51**: 165–169.

36. Cornoni-Huntley JC, Harris TB, Everett DF, Albanes D, Micozzi MS, Miles TP, Feldman JJ. An overview of body weight of older persons, including the impact on mortality: The National Health and Nutrition Examination Survey I—Epidemiologic follow-up study. *J Clin Epidemiol* 1991; **44**: 743–753.

37. Patrick JM, Bassey EJ, Fentem PH. Changes in body fat and muscle in manual workers at and after retirement. *Eur J Appl Physiol* 1982; **49**: 187–196.

38. Felson DT. Epidemiology of hip and knee osteoarthritis. *Epidemiol Rev* 1988; **10**: 1–28.

39. Campbell AJ, Spears GFS, Brown JS, Busby WJ, Borrie MJ. Anthropometric measurements as predictors of mortality in a community population aged 70 years and over. *Age Ageing* 1990; **19**: 131–135.

40. Ministry of Agriculture, Fisheries and Food. National Food Survey Committee. *Household food consumption and expenditure: 1987* Annual report of the National Food Survey Committee. London: HMSO, 1987.

41. Department of Health. *Dietary Sugars and Human Disease*. London: HMSO, 1989. (Reports on health and social subjects; 37).

42. Todd JE, Lader D. *Adult Dental Health 1988*. London: HMSO, 1991.

43. Carlsson GE. Masticatory efficiency: the effect of age, the loss of teeth and prosthetic rehabilitation. *Int Dent J* 1984; **34**: 93–97.

44. World Health Organization. *Diet, Nutrition, and the Prevention of Chronic Diseases. Report of a WHO Study Group*. Geneva: World Health Organization, 1990. (WHO Technical Report Series; 797).

45. Cummings JH, Bingham SA. Towards a recommended intake of dietary fibre. In: Eastwood M, Edwards C, Parry D, eds. *Human Nutrition: a continuing debate: Symposium entitled "Nutrition in the Nineties"*. London: Chapman & Hall, 1992; 107–108.

46. Uauy R, Winterer JC, Bilmazes C, Haverberg LN, Scrimshaw NS, Munro HN, Young VR. The changing pattern of whole body protein metabolism in ageing humans. *J Gerontol* 1978; **33**: 663–671.

47. Golden MHN, Waterlow JC. Total protein synthesis in elderly people; A comparison of results with ^{15}N glycine and ^{14}C leucine. *Clin Sci Mol Med* 1977; **53**: 277–288.

48. Lehmann AB, Johnston C, James OFW. The effects of old age and immobility on protein turnover in human subjects with some observations on the possible role of hormones. *Age Ageing* 1989; **18**: 148–157.

49. Gersovitz M, Motil K, Munro HN, Scrimshaw NS, Young VR. Human protein requirements: assessment of the adequacy of the current recommended allowance for dietary protein in elderly men and women. *Am J Clin Nutr* 1982; **35**: 6–14.

50. Reeds PJ, James WPT. Protein turnover. *Lancet* 1983; **I**: 571–574.

51. Rennie M, Harrison R. Effect of injury, disease and malnutrition on protein metabolism in man. Unanswered questions. *Lancet* 1984; **I**: 323–325.

52. Beaumont D, Lehmann AB, James OFW. Protein turnover in malnourished elderly subjects: the effect of refeeding. *Age Ageing* 1989; **18**: 235–240.

53. Zanni E, Calloway DH, Zezulka AY. Protein requirements of elderly men. *J Nutr* 1979; **109**: 513–524.

54. Willett WC. Vitamin A and lung cancer. *Nutr Rev* 1990; **48**: 201–211.

55. Bowman BB, Rosenberg IH. Assessment of the nutritional status of the elderly. *Am J Clin Nutr* 1982; **35**: 1142–1151.

56. Department of Health. *The Fortification of Yellow Fats with Vitamins A and D*. London: HMSO, 1991. (Reports on health and social subjects; 40).

57. Vir SC, Love AHG. Nutritional status of institutionalized aged in Belfast, Northern Ireland. *Am J Clin Nutr* 1979; **32**: 1934–1947.

58. Thomas AJ, Finglas P, Bunker VW. The B vitamin content of hospital meals and potential low intake by elderly inpatients. *J Hum Nutr Diet* 1988; **1**: 309–320.

59. O'Rourke NP, Bunker VW, Thomas AJ, Finglas PM, Bailey AL, Clayton BE. Thiamine status of healthy and institutionalized elderly subjects: analysis of dietary intake and biochemical indices. *Age Ageing* 1990; **19**: 325–329.

60. Sauberlich HE. Interactions of thiamin, riboflavin and other B vitamins. *Ann N Y Acad Sci* 1980; **355**: 80–97.

61. Older MJW, Dickerson JWT. Thiamine and the elderly orthopaedic patient. *Age Ageing* 1982; **11**: 101–107.

62. Thurnham D. Vitamins. In: Exton Smith A, Caird F, eds. *Metabolic and Nutritional Disorders in the Elderly*. Bristol: John Wright and Sons, 1980; 29–35.

63. Rutishauser IHE, Bates CJ, Paul AA, Black AE, Mandal AR, Patnaik BK. Long term vitamin status and dietary intake of healthy elderly subjects. *Br J Nutr* 1979; **42**: 33–42.

64. Chanarin I. *The Megaloblastic Anaemias*. London: Blackwell Scientific Publications, 1979; 315–354.

65. Suter PM, Russell RM, Vitamin requirements of the elderly. *Am J Clin Nutr* 1987; **45**: 501–512.

66. McEvoy AW, Fenwick JD, Boddy K, James OFW. Vitamin B_{12} absorption from the gut does not decline with age in normal elderly humans. *Age Ageing* 1982; **11**: 180–183.

67. Hitzhusen JC, Taplon ME, Stephenson WP, Ansell JE. Vitamin B_{12} levels and age. *Am J Clin Path* 1986; **85**: 32–36.

68. Hughes D, Elwood PC, Shinton NK, Wrighton RJ. Clinical trial of the effect of vitamin B_{12} in elderly subjects with low serum B_{12} levels. *BMJ* 1970; **1**: 458–460.

69. Waters WE, Withey JL, Kilpatrick GS, Wood PNH. Serum vitamin B_{12} concentrations in the general population—a ten year follow up. *Br J Haematol* 1971; **20**: 521–526.

70. Melamed E, Reches A, Herschko C. Reversible central nervous system dysfunction in folate deficiency. *J Neurolog Sci* 1975; **25**: 93–98.

71. Elwood PC, Shinton NK, Wilson CI, Sweetman P, Frazer AL. Haemoglobin vitamin B_{12} and folate levels in the elderly. *Br J Haematol* 1971; **21**: 557–563.

72. Webster SGP, Leeming JT. Erythrocyte folate levels in young and old. *J Am Geriat Soc* 1979; **27**: 451–454.

73. Girdwood RH, Thomson AD, Williamson J. Folate status in the elderly. *BMJ* 1967; **ii**: 670–672.

74. Blundell EL, Matthews JH, Allen SM, Middleton AM, Morris JE, Wickramasinghe SN. Importance of low serum B_{12} and red cell folate concentrations in elderly hospital inpatients. *J Clin Path* 1985; **38**: 1179–1184.

75. Stanton BR. *Meals for the elderly*. London: King Edwards's Hospital Fund for London, 1971.

76. Fenton J. Some food for thought. *Health Serv J* 1989; **99**: 666–667.

77. Schorah CJ. Inappropriate Vitamin C reserves. In: Taylor T et al eds. *The Importance of Vitamins to Human Health*. Lancaster: MTP Press, 1979; 61–72.

78. Gerster H. Review: Antioxidant protection of the ageing macula. *Age Ageing* 1991; **20**: 60–69.

79. Chandra RK. The relation between immunology, nutrition and disease in elderly people. *Age Ageing* 1990; **19**: S25–31.

80. Meydani SN, Blumberg JB. Nutrition and immune function in the elderly. In: Munro HN, Danford DE, eds. *Nutrition, Aging, and the Elderly*. New York: Plenum Press, 1989; 61–87.

81. Schultz BM, Freedman ML. Iron deficiency in the elderly. *Clinical Haematology* 1987; **1**: 291–313.

82. Finch CA. Nutritional Anaemia. In: Horwitz A, et al, eds. *Nutrition in the Elderly*. Oxford: Oxford University Press, 1989; 194–200.

83. Marx JJM. Normal iron absorption and decreased red-cell iron uptake in the aged. *Blood* 1979; **53**: 204–211.

84. Russell RM. Malabsorption and Ageing. In: Bianchi L *et al*, ed. *Ageing in Liver and Gastro-Intestinal Tract: 47th Falk Symposium*. Lancaster: Kluwer Academic, 1988; 297–308.

85. Thomas AJ, Bunker VW, Stansfield MF, Sodha NK, Clayton BE. Iron status of hospitalized and housebound elderly people. *Q J Med* 1989; **70**: 175–184.

86. Thomas AJ, Bunker VW, Hinks LJ, Sodha N, Mullee MA, Clayton BE. Energy, protein, zinc and copper status of twenty-one elderly in-patients: analysed dietary intake and biochemical indices. *Br J Nutr* 1988; **59**: 181–191.

87. Senapati A, Jenner G, Thompson RPH. Zinc in the elderly. *Q J Med* 1989; **70**: 81–87.

88. Chandra RK. Nutritional regulation of immunocompetence and risk of disease. In: Horwitz A *et al*, eds. *Nutrition in the Elderly*. Oxford: Oxford University Press, 1989; 203–218.

89. Wagner PA, Jernigan JA, Bailey LB, Nickens C, Brazzi GA. Zinc nutriture and cell mediated immunity in the aged. *Internat J Vit Nutr Res* 1983; **53**: 94–107.

90. Bogden JD, Oleske JM, Lavenhar MA, Munves EM, Kemp FW, Bruening KS, Holding KJ, Denny TN, Guarino MA, Krieger LM, Holland BK. Zinc and immunocompetence in elderly people: effect of zinc supplementation for 3 months. *Am J Clin Nutr* 1988; **48**: 655–663.

91. Moore R. Bleeding gastric erosion after zinc sulphate. *BMJ* 1978; **1**: 754.

92. Hoffman HN, Phyliky RL, Fleming CR. Zinc induced copper deficiency. *Gastroenterol* 1988; **94**: 508–512.

93. Nutritional copper status and catecholamine metabolism. *Nutr Rev* 1990; **48**: 416–418.

94. Sandstead HH. Copper bioavailability and requirements. *Am J Clin Nutr* 1982; **35**: 809–814.

95. Salonen JT, Salonen R, Lappetelainen R, Maenpaa PH, Alfthan G, Puska P. Risk of cancer in relation to serum concentrations of selenium and vitamins A and E: matched case control analysis of prospective data. *BMJ* 1985; **290**: 417–420.

96. Morley JE. The role of nutrition in the prevention of age associated diseases. In: Morley J, Glick Z, Rubenstein L, eds. *Geriatric Nutrition: a Comprehensive Review*. New York: Raven Press, 1990; 89–103.

97. Department of Health. *The Health of the Nation*. London: HMSO, 1992.

98. Cashin-Hemphill L, Mack WJ, Pogoda JM, Sanmarco ME, Azen SP, Blankenhorn DH. Beneficial effects of Colestipol-Niacin on coronary atherosclerosis. A 4-year follow-up. *J Am Med Assoc* 1990; **264**: 3013–3017.

99. Gofman JW, Young W, Tandy R. Ischemic heart disease, atherosclerosis and longevity. *Circulation* 1966; **34**: 679–697.

100. Gordon DJ, Rifkind BM. Treating high blood cholesterol in the older patient. *Am J Cardiol* 1989; **63**: 48H–52H.

101. Barrett-Connor E, Suarez L, Khaw K-T, Criqui MH, Wingard DL. Ischemic heart disease risk factors after age 50. *J Chron Dis* 1984; **37**: 903–908.

102. Shipley MJ, Pocock SJ, Marmot MG. Does plasma cholesterol concentration predict mortality from coronary heart disease in elderly people? 18 year follow-up in Whitehall study. *BMJ* 1991; **303**: 89–92.

103. Esterbauer H, Dieber-Rotheneder M, Striegl G, Waeg G. Role of vitamin E in preventing the oxidation of low-density lipoproteins. *Am J Clin Nutr* 1991; **53**: 314S–321S.

104. Fuster V, Badimon L, Badimon JJ, Cheesebro JH. The pathogenesis of coronary artery disease and the acute coronary syndromes. *N Engl J Med* 1992; **326**: 242–250.

105. The British Nutrition Foundation. *Unsaturated fatty acids. Nutritional and physiological significance*. Report of the British Nutrition Foundation's Task Force. London: The British Nutrition Foundation, 1992.

106. Williams RS. Logue EE, Lewis JL, Barton T, Stead NW, Wallace AG, Pizzo SV. Physical conditioning augments the fibrinolytic response to venous occlusion in healthy adults. *N Engl J Med* 1980; **302**: 987–991.

107. Morris JN, Clayton DG, Everitt MG, Semmence AM, Burgess EH. Exercise in leisure time: coronary attack and death rates. *Br Heart J* 1990; **63**: 325–334.

108. Intersalt Cooperative Research Group. Intersalt: an international study of electrolyte excretion and blood pressure. Results for 24 hour urinary sodium and potassium excretion. *BMJ* 1988; **297**: 319–328.

109. Law MR, Frost CD, Wald NJ. By how much does dietary salt reduction lower blood pressure? *BMJ* 1991; **302**: 811–824.

110. Grobbee DE, Hofman A. Does sodium restriction lower blood pressure? *BMJ* 1986; **293**: 27–29.

111. Krishna CG, Miller E, Kapoor S. Increased blood pressure during potassium depletion in normotensive men. *New Engl J Med* 1989; **320**: 1177–1182.

112. Boegehold MA, Kotchen TA. Relative contributions of dietary Na + and Cl − to salt-sensitive hypertension. *Hypertension* 1989; **14**: 579–583.

113. Forte JG, Miguel JMP, Miguel MJP, de Padua F, Rose G. Salt and blood pressure: a community trial. *J Hum Hypertension* 1989; **3**: 179–184.

114. Spector TD, Cooper C, Fenton Lewis A. Trends in admissions for hip fracture in England and Wales, 1968–85. *BMJ* 1990; **300**: 1173–1174.

115. Griffin J. *Osteoporosis and the Risk of Fracture*. London: Office of Health Economics, 1990. (Papers on current health problems No 94)

116. Kanders B, Dempster DW, Lindsay R. Interaction of calcium nutrition and physical activity on bone mass in young people. *J Bone Min Res* 1988; **3**: 145–149.

117. Riggs BL, Wahner HW, Melton LF III, Richelson LS, Judd HL, O'Fallon WM. Dietary calcium intake and rates of bone loss in women. *J Clin Invest* 1987; **80**: 979–982.

118. Stevenson JC, Whitehead MI, Padwick M, Endacott JA, Sutton C, Banks LM, Freemantle C, Spinks TJ, Hesp R. Dietary intake of calcium and postmenopausal bone loss. *BMJ* 1988; **297**: 15–17.

119. Matkovic V, Kostial K, Simonovic I, Buzina R, Brodarec A, Nordin BEC. Bone status and fracture rate in two regions of Yugoslavia. *Am J Clin Nutr* 1979; **32**: 540–549.

120. Holbrook TL, Barrett-Connor E, Wingard DL. Dietary calcium and risk of hip fracture: 14 year prospective population study. *Lancet* 1988; **ii**: 1046–1049.

121. Wooton R, Brereton PJ, Clark MB, Hesp R, Hodkinson HM, Klenerman L. Fractured neck of femur in the elderly: an attempt to identify patients at risk. *Clin Sci* 1979; **57**: 93–101.

122. Whickam CAC, Walsh K, Cooper C, Barker DJP, Margetts DH, Morris J, Bruce CA. Dietary calcium, physical activity and risk of hip fracture: a prospective study. *BMJ* 1989; **299**: 889–892.

123. Heaney RP, Recker RR, Saville PD. Menopausal changes in calcium balance performance. *J Lab Clin Med* 1978; **92**: 953–963.

124. Francis RM, Peacock M, Storer JH, Davies AEJ, Brown WB, Nordin BEC. Calcium malabsorption in the elderly; the effect of treatment with oral 25-hydroxyvitamin D. *Eur J Clin Invest* 1983; **13**: 391–396.

125. Francis RM, Peacock M, Barkworth SA. Renal impairment and its effects on calcium metabolism in elderly women. *Age Ageing* 1984; **13**: 14–20.

126. Nordin BEC, Baker MR, Horsman A, Peacock M. A prospective trial of the effect of vitamin D supplementation on metacarpal bone loss in elderly women. *Am J Clin Nutr* 1985; **42**: 470–474.

127. Bunker VW, Lawson MS, Stansfield MF, Clayton BE. The intake and excretion of calcium, magnesium and phosphorus in apparently healthy elderly people and those who are housebound. *J Clin Exp Gerontol* 1989; **11**: 71–86.

128. Ministry of Agriculture, Fisheries and Food. National Food Survey Committee. *Household food consumption and expenditure: 1975, 1990.* Annual reports of the National Food Survey Committee. London: HMSO, 1976, 1991.

129. National Dairy Council. *Liquid Milk Report 1991.* London: National Dairy Council, 1991.

130. Lawson DEM, Paul AA, Black AE, Cole TJ, Mandal AR, Davie M. Relative contributions of diet and sunlight to vitamin D state in the elderly. *BMJ* 1979; **2**: 303–305.

131. Francis RM. The pathogenesis of osteoporosis. In: Francis R, ed. *Osteoporosis: Pathogenesis and Management.* Lancaster: Kluwer Academic, 1990; 51–80.

132. Lips P, Wiersinga A, van Ginkel FC, Jongen MJM, Netelenbos JC, Hackeng WHL, Delmas PD, van der Vijgn WJF. The effect of vitamin D supplementation on vitamin D status and parathyroid function in elderly subjects. *J Clin Endocrin Metabol* 1988; **67**: 644–650.

133. Aaron JE, Gallagher JC, Anderson J, Stasiak L, Longton EB, Nordin BEC, Nicholson M. Frequency of osteomalacia in fractures of the proximal femur. *Lancet* 1974; **i**: 229–233.

134. Hordon LD, Peacock M. Osteomalacia and osteoporosis in femoral neck fracture. *Bone Mineral* 1990; **11**: 247–259.

135. Compston JE, Vedi S, Croucher PI. Low prevalence of osteomalacia in elderly patients with hip fracture. *Age Ageing* 1991; **20**: 132–134.

136. Holick MF. The intimate relationship between the sun, skin and vitamin D: a new perspective. Bone: *Clinical and Biochemical News and Reviews* 1990; **7**: 66–69.

137. Department of Health and Social Security. *Rickets and Osteomalacia.* London: HMSO, 1980. (Reports on health and social subjects; 19)

138. Chalmers J. Vitamin D deficiency in elderly people. *BMJ* 1991; **303**: 314–315.

139. Krall EA, Sahyoun N, Tannenbaum S, Dallal GE, Dawson-Hughes B. Effect of vitamin D intake on seasonal variations in parathyroid hormone secretion in postmenopausal women. *N Engl J Med* 1989; **321**: 1777–1783.

140. Dawson-Hughes B, Dallas GE, Krall EA, Harris S, Sokoll LJ, Fakoner C. Effect of vitamin D supplementation on wintertime and overall bone loss in healthy postmenopausal women. *Ann Int Med* 1991; **115**: 505–512.

141. Davies M, Mawer EB, Hann JT, Stephens WP, Taylor JL. Vitamin D prophylaxis in the elderly; a simple effective method suitable for large populations. *Age Ageing* 1985; **14**: 349–354.

142. Bernstein PS, Sadowsky N, Hegsted DM, Guri CD, Stave FJ. Prevalence of osteoporosis in high and low fluoride areas in North Dakota. *J Am Med Assoc* 1966; **198**: 499–504.

143. Alffram PA, Hernborg J, Nillson BER. The influence of a high fluoride content in the drinking water on the bone mineral mass in man. *Acta Orthop Scand* 1969; **40**: 137–142.

144. Simonen O, Laitinen O. Does fluoridation of drinking-water prevent bone fragility and osteoporosis? *Lancet* 1985; **ii**: 432–433.

145. Riggs BL, Hodgson SF, O'Fallon M, Chao EYS, Wahner HW, Muhs JM, Cedel SL, Melton LJ. Effects of fluoride treatment on the fracture rate in postmenopausal women with osteoporosis. *New Engl J Med* 1990; **322**, 802–809.

146. Office of Population Censuses and Surveys. *Cancer Statistics Registrations England and Wales 1986*. Series MB1 No 19. London: HMSO, 1991.

147. Doll R, Peto R. *The Causes of Cancer*. Oxford: Oxford University Press, 1981.

148. Linn BS, Linn MS. Dietary patterns and practices which affect the incidence of cancer in the elderly. In: Watson R, ed. *Handbook of Nutrition in the Aged*. Boca Raton, F1: CRC press, 1985; 299–311.

149. Colditz GA, Branch LG, Lipnick KJ. Increased green and yellow vegetable intake and lowered cancer deaths in an elderly population. *Am J Clin Nutr* 1985; **41**: 32–36.

150. Thurnham DI. Antioxidants and pro-oxidants in malnourished populations. *Proc Nut Soc* 1990; **45**: 247–259.

151. Morgan BD, Newton HMV, Schorah CJ, Jewitt MA, Hancock MR, Hullin RP. Abnormal indices of nutrition in the elderly: a study of different clinical groups. *Age Ageing* 1986; **15**: 65–76.

152. Sandstrom B, Alhaug J, Einarsdottir K, Simpura EM, Isaksson B. Nutritional status, energy and protein intake in general medical patients in three Nordic hospitals. *Hum Nutr: Appl Nutr* 1985; **39A**: 87–94.

153. Barnes KE. *The Interaction of Nutrition and Nursing Care in Elderly, Longstay Patients.* London: University of London (UCL), 1988. PhD Thesis.

154. Elmstahl S, Steen B. Hospital nutrition in geriatric long term care medicine: II. Effects of dietary supplements. *Age Ageing* 1987; **16**: 73-80.

155. Levi S, Cox M, Lugon M, Hodkinson M, Tomkins A. Increased energy expenditure in Parkinson's disease. *BMJ* 1990; **301**: 1256-1257.

156. Sandman PO, Adofsson R, Nygren C, Hallmans G, Winblad B. Nutritional status and dietary intake in institutionalized patients with Alzheimer's disease and multiinfarct dementia. *J Am Geriatr Soc* 1987; **35**: 31-38.

157. Prentice AM, Leavesley K, Murgatroyd PR, Coward WA, Schorah CJ, Bladon PT, Hullin RP. Is severe wasting in elderly mental patients caused by an excessive energy requirement? *Age Ageing* 1989; **18**: 158-167.

158. Ximenes R, Cox M, Tomkins AM, Collins K. Energy expenditure in vaccination infection and controlled hyperthermia. *Proc Nutr Soc* 1987; **46**: 16A.

159. Cox ML, Rudd AG, Gallimore R, Hodkinson HM, Pepys MB. Realtime measurement of serum C-reactive protein in the management of infection in the elderly. *Age Ageing* 1986; **15**: 257-266.

160. Hodkinson HM, Cox M, Lugon M, Cox ML, Tomkins A. Energy cost of chest infections in the elderly. *J Clin Exper Gerontol* 1990; **12**: 241-246.

161. Bistrian BR. Blackburn GL, Hallowell E, Heddle R. Protein status of general surgical patients. *J Am Med Assoc* 1974; **230**: 858-860.

162. Klidjian AM, Foster KJ, Kammerling RM, Cooper A, Karran SJ. Relation of anthropometric and dynamometric variables to serious postoperative complications. *BMJ* 1980; **281**: 899 901.

163. Hill GL, Pickford I, Young GA, Schorah CJ, Blackett RL, Burkinshaw L, Warren JV, Morgan DB. Malnutrition in surgical patients: an unrecognised problem. *Lancet* 1977; **I**: 689-692.

164. Kemm JR, Allcock J. The distribution of supposed indicators of nutritional status in elderly patients. *Age Ageing* 1984; **13**: 21-28.

165. Ford MG, Neville JN. Nutritive intake of nursing home patients served three or five meals a day. *J Am Diet Assoc* 1972; **61**: 292-296.

166. Suski NS, Nielson CC. Factors affecting food intake of women with Alzheimer's type dementia in long-term care. *J Am Diet Assoc* 1989; **89**: 1770-1773.

167. Bastow MD, Rawlings J, Allison SP. Benefits of supplementary tube feeding after fractured neck of femur: a randomised controlled trial. *BMJ* 1983; **287**: 1589-1592.

168. Delmi M, Rapin CH, Bengoa JM, Delmas PD, Vasey H, Bonjour JP. Dietary supplementation in elderly patients with fractured neck of the femur. *Lancet* 1990; **335**: 1013–1016.

169. Katakity M, Webb JF, Dickerson JWT. Some effects of a food supplement in elderly hospital patients: A longitudinal study. *Hum Nutr: Appl Nutr* 1983; **37A**: 85–93.

170. Banerjee AK, Brocklehurst JC, Wainwright H, Swindell R. Nutritional status of long-stay geriatric in-patients: Effects of a food supplement (Complan). *Age Ageing* 1978; **7**: 237–243.

171. Williams CM, Driver LT, Older J, Dickerson J. A controlled trial of sip-feed supplements in elderly orthopaedic patients. *Eur J Clin Nutr* 1989; **43**: 267–274.

Annex 1. Dietary Reference Values for food energy and nutrients for people aged over 50 years in the United Kingdom.

In 1991 the UK government published Dietary Reference Values for energy and nutrient intakes for the United Kingdom[1]. The figures rest on a value for the *Estimated Average Requirement* (EAR). The *Reference Nutrient Intake* (RNI) is the daily amount sufficient, or more than sufficient, to meet the nutritional needs of practically all healthy persons in a population and therefore exceeds the requirements of most. The value is set at a notional 2 standard deviations above the EAR for each nutrient. Energy requirements are given only as the average for a population group. The EAR for energy per day for adults is shown in Table 4.1. The EAR and RNI for vitamins and minerals are given in tables A1 and A2. The recommendations of the COMA Panel on DRV concerning macronutrients are described in the text of the present report.

Reference

[1] Department of Health. *Dietary Reference Values for Food Energy and Nutrients for the United Kingdom*. London: HMSO, 1991. (Reports on health and social subjects; 41).

Table A1: *Dietary Reference Values for vitamins for people aged 50 + years in the United Kingdom*

	male		female	
	EAR	RNI	EAR	RNI
Thiamin (mg/1000 kcal/d)	0.3	0.4	0.3	0.4
Riboflavin (mg/d)	1.0	1.3	0.9	1.1
Niacin (mg/d)	13	16	10	12
Vitamin B_6 (μg/g/d protein)	0.7	1.4	0.6	1.2
Vitamin B_{12} (μg/d)	1.25	1.5	1.25	1.5
Folate (μg/d)	150	200	150	200
Vitamin C (mg/d)	25	40	25	40
Vitamin A (μg/d retinol equivalent)	500	700	400	700
Vitamin D (μg/d)	*	10**	*	10**

*EAR not set   **for population aged 65 years or more only

Table A2: *Dietary Reference Values for minerals for people aged 50 + years in the United Kingdom*

	male				female			
	EAR		RNI		EAR		RNI	
Calcium mmol(mg/d)	13.1	(525)	17.5	(700)	13.1	(525)	17.5	(700)
Phosphorus mmol(mg/d)	13.1	(400)	17.5	(550)	13.1	(400)	17.5	(550)
Magnesium mmol(mg/d)	10.3	(250)	12.3	(300)	8.2	(200)	10.9	(270)
Sodium mmol(mg/d)	*		70	(1600)	*		70	(1600)
Potassium mmol(mg/d)	*		90	(3500)	*		90	(3500)
Chloride mmol(mg)	*		70	(2500)	*		70	(2500)
Iron μmol(mg/d)	120	(6.7)	160	(8.7)	120	(6.7)	160	(8.7)
Zinc μmol(mg/d)	110	(7.3)	145	(9.5)	85	(5.5)	110	(7.0)
Copper μmol(mg/d)	*		19	(1.2)	*		19	(1.2)
Selenium μmol(μg/d)	*		0.9	(75)	*		0.8	(60)
Iodine μmol(mg/d)	*		1.1	(140)	*		1.1	(140)

*No EAR set

Annex 2. Methods of measuring body composition with a comment on the applicability of the method for use with elderly people

INDIRECT METHODS

Commonly used indirect methods of body mass index and skinfold thickness are considered in section 5.3.

Bio-electric impedance or total body conductivity The electrical impedance or conductance of the body is related to the proportions of fat and lean tissue[1]. Various empirical equations have been derived by comparing the results with those obtained using established methods. The equations for elderly people differ from those found for younger adults and this is presumed to be due to variations in the concentrations of body fluids in the intra- and extra-cellular compartments. These equations have been validated in a group aged over 65 years against underwater weighing with direct assessment of residual volume; the estimates of fat free mass had a standard error of the mean of $\pm$ 2.5 kg[2]. The method is relatively cheap, convenient, non-invasive and requires no special skills and may be particularly valuable in elderly people.

Ultrasound Scanning B-mode scanning allows the measurement of the thickness of fat plus skin at specific body sites. The ultrasound beam reflects off the tissue interface and the phase change in the beam can be used to assess the depth of the interface from the surface. It is not widely used for assessing fat except in animal husbandry. It has many of the disadvantages of skinfold measurements whilst being more expensive, and cumbersome.

Near infra-red interactance This is a relatively new technique which was also developed for animal husbandry. It depends on transmission through the body of infra-red radiation at two wavelengths and the selective effects on that transmission of fat and lean tissue. The shift in the wavelengths is related to the amount of fat and lean tissue in the path of the beam. The radiation is harmless. It has been validated in humans against underwater weighing and isotope dilution in body water but not in elderly people. It has been found to underestimate fat systematically but may nevertheless be a useful approach[3].

DIRECT METHODS

Underwater weighing Estimates of body density obtained by underwater weighing can be used to calculate the percentage of fat and lean tissue. This method is often used as a standard against which to validate other methods, however it also depends on assumptions. Fixed values for the densities of fat, bone and fat-free mass are used, and a fixed proportion of fat-free mass is assumed to be bone[4]. These assumptions may not be valid for elderly people, for instance, osteoporotic subjects have less dense bones, so an over-estimate of fat is made. Furthermore, intra-abdominal gas causes an under-estimate of density and therefore an over-estimate of fat. Gas in the lungs has to be measured or estimated from height and age. Only the most robust people are willing to submerge themselves completely and then perform the re-breathing manoeuvres which are necessary to obtain the residual volume. In an age group in which lung disease causes wide variation in residual volume, there will be under estimation of the residual volume if predictions are made from data for young healthy lungs and this leads to an over-estimation of the fat.

Total body potassium   The natural gamma radiation from the small amount of isotopic body potassium can be used to assess lean body mass non-invasively since almost all the potassium is in this compartment[5]. The technique is expensive, it requires sensitive gamma counters situated in an environment which is free from confounding sources of natural radiation. Elderly people have a lower lean body mass than younger adults and so need more sensitive equipment or a longer period of counting. Lying alone on a hard surface in a strange environment is not well tolerated by frail elderly individuals and this method is not suitable for routine use.

Neutron activation   Gamma rays are emitted from nitrogen and hydrogen nuclei in the body when they are bombarded with neutrons. Gamma counters (see above) can then be used to assess the amount of these constituents[6]. From this information total body protein or lean mass can be calculated from standard conversion factors. This is also expensive and unsuitable for routine use.

DILUTION METHODS

Deuterium or tritium dilution   Total body water can be assessed using the dilution space of the stable isotope deuterium or the radio-active isotope tritium which has a convenient half-life of a few hours. It has to be assumed that the label can reach all non-fat compartments[7] and care must be taken to account for water lost from the body and that produced by metabolism during the equilibration period[8]. Assumptions are then made about the specific gravity of lean tissue and the proportion of bone in order to convert the water volume into lean mass and so partition the body into fat and lean compartments. The technique requires a mass spectrometer and expensive isotopes. It promises to be useful but it has not yet been validated for elderly people.

SCANNING

Absorptiometric scanning techniques   Computerised scanning techniques can be used to image bone, fat and lean tissue because the tissues absorb photons differentially[9]. Computer x-ray tomography has been in use for some time for body segments such as the thigh. However, the radiation dose is unacceptably high for repeated use and the technique is expensive. More recently photon sources with dual energy levels have been used to image the body and assess the fat and lean components as well as bone with a reliability of ± 1.5 per cent[10,11]. Gadolinium has been used as the photon source but the running costs are high and calibration problems can occur when the Gd source is renewed. It is now possible to use low dose dual energy X-ray machines as the photon source with a precision of ± 1.0 per cent. It is likely that this may become a reference technique against which other techniques such as impedance can be validated.

References

1 Lukaski HC, Bolonchuk WW, Hall CB, Siders WA. Validation of tetrapolar bioelectrical impedance method to assess human body composition. *J Appl Physiol* 1986; **60**: 1327–1332.

2 Deurenberg P, Van der Kooij K, Evers P, Hulshof T. Assessment of body composition by bioelectrical impedance in a population aged >60 y. *Am J Clin Nutr* 1990; **51**: 3–6.

3 Conway JM, Norris KH, Bodwell CE. A new approach for the estimation of body composition: infrared interactance. *Am J Clin Nutr* 1984; **40**: 1123–1130.

4 Siri WE. *Body composition from fluid spaces and density: analysis of methods*. University of California Radiation Laboratory Report 1956; 3349.

5 Bruce A, Andersson M, Arvidsson B, Isaksson B. Body composition. Prediction of normal body potassium, body water and body fat in adults on the basis of body height, body weight and age. *Scand J Clin Lab Invest* 1980; **40**: 461–473.

6 Vartsky D, Ellis KJ, Cohn SH. In vivo quantification of body nitrogen by analysis of prompt gammas from neutron capture. *J Nucl Med* 1979; **20**: 1158–1165.

7 Schoeller DA, van Santen E, Peterson DW, Dietz W, Jaspan J, Klein PD. Total body water measurement in humans with ^{18}O and ^{2}H labelled water. *Am J Clin Nutr* 1980; **33**: 2686–2693.

8 Roberts SB. Use of the doubly labelled water method for measurement of energy expenditure, total body water, water intake, and metabolizable energy intake in humans and small animals. *Can J Physiol Pharmacol* 1989; **67**: 1190–1198.

9 Young A, Stokes M, Crowe M. Size and strength of the quadriceps muscles of old and young women. *Eur J Clin Invest* 1984; **14**: 282–287.

10 Gotfredsen A, Jensen J, Borg J, Christiansen C. Measurement of lean body mass and total body fat using dual photon absorptiometry. *Metabolism* 1986; **35**: 88–93.

11 Heymsfield SB, Lichtman S, Baumgartner RN, Wang J, Kamen Y, Aliprantis A, Pierson R. Body composition of humans: comparison of two improved four-compartment models that differ in expense, technical complexity, and radiation exposure. *Am J Clin Nutr* 1990; **52**: 52–58.

Annex 3. Register of members' commercial interests

Professor H M Hodkinson (Chairman)

Personal interests: None
Non-personal interests: None

Professor J Grimley Evans

Personal interests: None
Non-personal interests: None

Dr R M Francis

Personal interests: None
Non-personal interests:

Sandoz	Commissioned Research Work
Leo	,,
Sanofi	,,
Merck, Sharp and Dohme	,,
Norwich Eaton	,,
Duphar	,,
Smith, Kline, Beechams	,,
Rorer	,,
Leo Foundation	Research grant

Professor O F W James

Personal interests: None
Non-personal interests: None

Professor W P T James

Personal interests: None
Non-personal interests:

Fisons	Research support

Dr K E Jones

Personal interests: None
Non-personal interests: None

Professor A J Thomas

Personal interests: None
Non-personal interests: None

Index

Printed in the United Kingdom for HMSO
Dd300771 2/95 C5 G559 10170